CONTENTS

INTRODUCTION

Many people of all ages suffer from stiffness and mobility issues. Movement is at the base of being alive; we can't get away from it, which is why it is so important to be able to do it with ease. When people suffer from persistent stiff muscles or pain during movement, they usually attribute it to age, injury, or something else that they cannot control. Maybe those things can play a factor, but lack of flexibility is the number one cause of stiff muscles and pain.

If you suffer from constant injuries while training, hindered movement due to muscle stiffness, or pain, then you may have a flexibility issue. The good news is that you do not have to suffer from this forever; flexibility is something that you can gain over time. What you need is a tailor-made set of stretches and flexibility exercises that will help you increase your mobility. Not all stretches are created equal, and some only work for specific needs and circumstances, that is why just doing generic stretches will not work. The road to flexibility and increased mobility is a journey that you need to be guided along so that you can get the best out of it.

After years of experience as a personal trainer and physio, I have confronted every reason for inflexibility in the book. Because of this, I have been able to devise tailored solutions to various problems. I take pride in my ability to help people along this journey and am confident that I will be able to help you. Being able to reach a place where your body can have its full range of motion with no pain or stiffness is life-altering. All it takes is a few simple routines and consistency, and I know you will be able to reach the level of flexibility you once were and even exceed that.

My clients are now enjoying their lives much more; they did not know how free life could be until they were able to remove the constraints that their bodies had. They are much happier, and they can reach their fitness goals much quicker, training is no longer a chore but rather a joy to do. With a little effort, you can also have a similar story. You will be able to touch your toes with ease, walk for hours with no pain, and take your training to the next level. Movement will no longer be an obstacle that is standing in your way, but the stepping stone you can use to reach your other goals.

This book will be filled with routines, tips, tricks, and knowledge I have passed on to my clients, who are now enjoying life to the full. They now know that nothing can stand in their way. They can push themselves more each day because they see what their bodies are capable of. Once they reached this realization, they became more confident in their bodies' capabilities, and that is what I want for everyone who reads through these pages.

By the time you are done with this book, you will be fully equipped with the knowledge that will help you gain back your flexibility or tap into the flexibility you never knew you had. Armed with stretches and routines that have been tailor-made for your circumstance means that you get to focus on what is best for you. It will cut out the frustration of trying lots of different things that just don't work. Everyone's body and circumstances are different, and that is why I have made sure that there is something for everyone in this book.

Until you make an effort to start working on your flexibility, stiff and sore muscles will always be an issue. In fact, the longer you do not address the problem, the worse it will get. Flexibility is not only about excelling in sports and fitness but also in your everyday life. Inflexibility can get in the way of doing simple tasks like bending down to fetch something from the cupboard or picking up your child or grandchild. The sooner you start, the sooner you can begin reaping the benefits. You will feel younger and be able to perform the tasks that now cause a problem, with ease.

The knowledge that I will be passing on to you has helped hundreds of people. They now live more nimble and pain-free lives, all because of the guidance provided in this book. Each chapter will provide you with the steps and support needed to make the most out of your potential mobility and say goodbye to your flexibility struggles. Applying what you learn will lead you to improve flexibility problems associated with pain and stiffness, so you no longer have to deal with it daily. Once you start feeling and seeing the results from utilizing the tools given to you in this book, you will never look back.

Your better, freer, and more mobile life is just on the other side of these pages. Once you start unlocking the potential that your body has, you will want to push forward and try new things. My goal is that everyone who reads this book will benefit in some way and, as a result, live a better life altogether. If you want to lose the inflexibility chains that have bound you for so long, then this is your first step. Let's go on this journey together.

1

THE WARM-UP: BENEFITS OF STRETCHING THAT YOU ARE MISSING OUT ON

S tretching is often overlooked when planning a workout program. Usually, people have goals like losing weight or gaining muscle, and they believe that stretching will not be of much help to them. This kind of thinking is incorrect; stretching is vital to every movement of your body. It allows your body to have the freedom to move as it pleases and reduces the amount of pain you will have when exerting pressure on your muscles.

THE IMPORTANCE OF STRETCHING

Stretching is not only a physical thing, but it also overflows in every part of your wellbeing. It will increase the level in which your body can move, improve your quality of life, even impact your mental wellbeing. It is what will empower your body to do the activities that will help you reach your body goals and can be used as a tool to calm your mind through life's ups and downs. What's even more impressive is that's just scratching the surface of how beneficial stretching can be to your life.

Exercise

Stretching is focused on lengthening the muscles, and it allows your muscles to function better. When you stretch, it improves your body's mobility, which is so essential to exercising. When you exercise, you are using your muscles, that's why you need them to be in top form. Increasing your range of mobility will benefit the way you exercise because you will not be restricted to tight muscles, you will be able to engage more muscles in your body and increase the quality of your workout.

Flexibility is sometimes not thought of as something linked to strength. This is entirely false, and if you don't believe me, just look at people who do yoga, both men and women alike have toned bodies and a significant amount of strength. Flexibility in itself is not strength training, but because your muscles work together in everything, you are able to get more out of your strength workouts when you are more flexible.

Stretching is not a warm-up, as we have popularly thought. The truth is that you will get better results from stretching if your muscles are already warmed up. The best thing you can do is do a quick five-minute jog or walk around the block to get your muscles moving, then begin stretching. Your muscles will be looser, and you will get more out of your stretching routine. If you would like you can move on to your other exercises, your muscles will be nice and limber. When we incorporate stretching into our routine, it almost guarantees a reduction in injuries when exercising or putting any strain on our muscles. Our muscles are less likely to seize up and move into different positions more easily.

General Living

The lives we live now are quite sedentary, meaning that we don't move around a lot. We end up sitting at desks for most of the day, the most mobile part of our body is our fingers which are typing away at the keyboard. This isn't good for our muscles; in fact, sitting on a chair for most of the day will definitely result in tighter hamstrings. Now I am not saying you have to quit your job and become a professional athlete to be healthy, but balance is needed to keep your body healthy.

This balance is found when incorporating stretching into your routine. Sometimes we get so caught up in our busy everyday routine that we forget to do what is good for us. If you have ever suffered from stiff joints and pain or stiffness in certain muscles, even when you don't remember doing anything that can cause that feeling, then you should know that this is a direct result of a lack of mobility in your muscles.

Mobility will help you to go about your daily tasks with ease. Not being able to bend down to get something from the floor or a low shelf because of stiff muscles is not the greatest feeling, and it gets in the way of you just living your life. A high-quality life is one with as little restrictions as possible, we all want the freedom to do as we please, and our bodies should not be the thing that holds us back from doing that. This is precisely why flexibility and mobility are essential.

As we get older, our muscles and joints naturally get stiffer. Increasing your flexibility by stretching actually slows down this process. Getting started today will have you saying thank you in the future. We all still want to be able to do the things that we enjoy; we don't want aging to stop us from enjoying our lives. The earlier you start, the better it will be for you. However, don't discount the benefits of stretching in older years, stretching will always have massive benefits for whoever does it, regardless of age.

A direct result of stretching is healthier and stronger muscles. When our muscles are strong, our posture also improves. Slouching is a common problem today, and it can cause pain in your neck and back, and in severe cases, it can even lead to fatigue and shortness of breath. When we stretch, it encourages the proper alignment of our muscles, which pulls our bodies up and reduces the risk of slouching and bad posture.

Another benefit of stretching is that it increases the blood circulation in our bodies. That means our bodies will be able to function better because of the increased blood supply to our muscles. With the increase in blood supply comes an increase in nutrients; this means the nutrient supply to our muscles is increased. You will also experience less soreness because of this increased blood and nutrient supply in your body. Your body will be able to function better as a whole.

Mental Wellbeing

During the day, our minds are so busy, always having problems to fix or a crisis to tend to. It is difficult to take the time to gather your thoughts and just focus on you. Not having time to clear your mind and focus on something that calms you can have negative impacts on your mental state. When you are always on the move, there is no time for rest, and we all need rest to perform our best. This rest should be both a physical as well as mental rest; we often overlook the latter.

When we stretch, it is a series of slow, controlled movements. We are forced to focus on ourselves, what our bodies are doing, and how we are feeling. This gives your mind a mental break from all the thoughts that are continually running through your mind. You have time to give your mind a break, destress, and begin to catch up with your thoughts. When you are done, you will feel more ready to take on the next set of challenges.

We can carry tension in our muscles; you will notice this in knots in your muscles, especially around your neck and shoulders. It is a defensive strategy used by our bodies when we are feeling stressed or overwhelmed. This can affect your performance throughout the day; you will be feeling uncomfortable and will always be thinking about the tension you are carrying in your muscles. Stretching provides a better outlet for this stress, not only that it can help with preventing knots in the future.

Stress and tension have a negative effect on our mental wellbeing. What goes on in our minds will eventually overflow into all other areas of life. Don't overlook how important mental health is to your overall health and happiness. We need to take care of all aspects of our wellbeing.

DO IT RIGHT

As much as it is important to start somewhere, we have to be doing things correctly. Granted, you will not be an expert at the beginning of this journey, but neglecting the proper way to stretch can cause more harm than good. It is essential to set your expectations at the beginning so that you are aware of what it entails and know how to get the best results. That's what I want for you, I want you to get the best possible results, and that is only achievable through moving forward in the right way.

The Right Form

The proper form refers to the right execution of each and every stretch; this will make sure you will get the best out of your stretching routine. Many stretching exercises focus on isolated muscle groups, so when you are stretching, you will know where you should feel it. Paying attention to where you feel the stretch and how you are stretching, in general, is a vital part of getting a good workout.

Stretching causes tension in your muscles, so when you feel this, you know that you are working on something. However, it should never cause pain. If you do feel pain, then that is an indication that you are doing something wrong or have stretched too far for your muscles at this point. As soon as you feel pain, stop, assess why there was pain, and try and avoid that in the future. The saying "no pain, no gain" does not apply in this situation. Pushing yourself too far might result in torn muscles and damage to the tissues.

Make sure you have the right amount of space for the stretch. You do not want to be in mid-stretch and then be stopped by a piece of furniture or the wall. In most cases, you cannot modify a stretch for a smaller space, so if you try, you might not even get the benefits of that stretch. Make sure you know how to do the stretch before you attempt it. This will help you plan better both in terms of space and form. Knowing where your body is going with help with smoother transitions and a better experience overall.

Stretches are held for about 30 seconds or more; this is to make sure that your body has tension in the muscle. Doing it for too little time might not have as much of an effect as taking your time. Stretching is not about speed but rather about control, so focus on controlling your movements; this will make you more conscious about how you are executing your movements. Do not rush in and out of stretches; use your breathing as a guide if you need to. Slowing down your breathing can help you to slow down your movement and have more control.

A helpful tip is to watch yourself in the mirror. This way, you can see how you look when doing the stretch and pick up if you're doing something wrong much easier. Check your form in the mirror, especially with new and more difficult stretches. Once you are more comfortable, you can move away from the mirror. If you do not have a mirror, try recording yourself. It has the same effect, but you do not have to be confined to a room with a mirror.

Getting your form and execution right is one of the most important things you can do. It will prevent injury and make sure that you are getting the best out of your stretches. This will reduce frustration since many people feel like they aren't getting anywhere, but this is just because they are not doing the stretches correctly. Once you learn how to perform the stretches correctly, half the battle is won. It will make the whole experience better and more worthwhile.

It Takes Time

Like with many things in life, stretching is all about consistency and effort. You won't suddenly become flexible after one or two stretching sessions; it takes time. Think about it, your body has not been flexible for your whole life, and now you are going to have to retrain your muscles. It might take a few months to start getting your flexibility, but it is all worth it, and hard work will pay off in the end.

You should be stretching every day, but if you cannot commit to this, then try for three to four times a week. If you do not do it often enough, then you might lose the flexibility you have gained, consistency is key. The amount of time that you spend on stretching for each session can vary depending on a few factors, but the important thing is to have a plan and then stick to it. Ten minutes of stretching every day will have greater benefits than two hours of stretching every other week. Remember, we are training our muscles to behave in a certain way.

Make it a routine, write it down somewhere so that you do not forget. Once you make it a priority, you are more likely to do it, and the more you do it, the better it will be for you. It will definitely help to plan out your stretching routine before you do it, you are more likely to stick to something if it is planned out. Plan it out a week in advance, know what you are doing for the whole week; that way, you just have to jump into the routine. This will help with consistency. I know all this seems obvious and trivial, but this is because people seriously do overlook the simple things, planning a stretching routine before they do it or making sure to do it for the full amount of time.

It might be hard in the beginning, the first time doing anything is hard, but keep at it and don't get discouraged. The results that await you on the other side is well worth the time and effort. Consistency always brings the greatest rewards.

MOBILITY AND FLEXIBILITY TEST

Mobility and flexibility go hand in hand, but they are not interchangeable, so it is crucial to work on both of them. Too much of one and not enough of the other could lead to injuries down the line. Bedosky (2018), shows us the difference between mobility and flexibility. Mobility deals with the joints and their range of movement, having excellent mobility means that you can move your joints through their full range of movement without any pain, discomfort, or restriction. Flexibility focuses on the lengthening of the muscles; good flexibility refers to being able to stretch and bend your muscles without restriction and tightness. Both of these take work to improve on, but they should be worked on together in order to get the best results.

We all need a place to start, and for us to start at the right place, we need actually to know what our current ability is. Elorreaga (2018) developed a mobility test that will help you determine where you are in terms of mobility and flexibility. This test is divided into sections depending on what part of the body is being focused on. Before you move forward in your journey, it is wise to do the test and see what you need to focus on more and why certain parts of your body are tight. I will take you through each assessment, which can all be done at home. This is not to replace any advice given by a doctor or physiotherapist; at the end of the day, I am not there with you, so if your qualified health professional has given you instruction or advice, then you should go with that. These assessments are designed to provide you with a benchmark for your mobility, but they do not diagnose any medical problems.

Our bodies will give us different results when it is warmed up and when our muscles are cold. Try and do these assessments once when your muscles are stiff, since that will give you an idea of your everyday mobility and flexibility. Then do it again when your muscles have warmed up, maybe after a workout so that you can compare.

You may be tempted to skip a few that you think you can easily do; I can assure you it's likely your mobility could shock you with how bad it is, so it is worth trying all moves to assess where your problem areas are.

UPPER BODY MOBILITY

The following movements will determine your mobility or flexibility in various upper body joints and muscles.

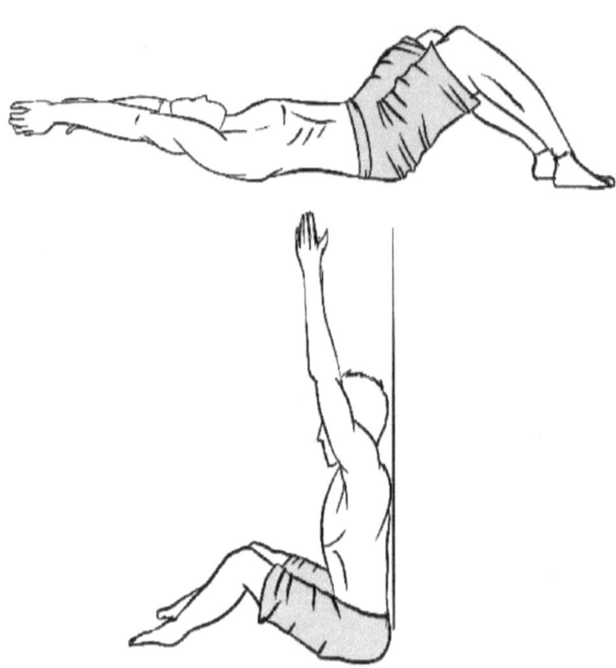

Shoulder Flexion

This move is designed to target your shoulder flexibility and mobility. It will show your ability to move your arms above your head at an increasing angle, away from your torso.

Flexibility Test Instructions:

- Lay on the ground, with the back flat.
- Raise your arms so that they move over your head.
- Your arms should lay flat on the ground behind you, without you having to arch your back.
- Your arms should not be bent, and your ribs should not be excessively flaring.

If you are unable to do this, then it indicates that you might have tight lats, pecs, biceps long head, rotator cuff, triceps, or a low thoracic extension. If you can do this, then you have excellent overhead flexibility.

Mobility Test Instructions:

- Sit with your back straight up against the wall.
- Same as the previous test, lift your arms so that they are above your head.
- They should be touching the wall without an arched back, bent arms, or flared rib cage.

If you are unable to do this and were able to do the previous test, then this indicates that you have low overhead mobility. You may suffer from weak or tight rotator cuffs, serratus anterior, or lower traps. If you were able to do this, then you have excellent overhead mobility.

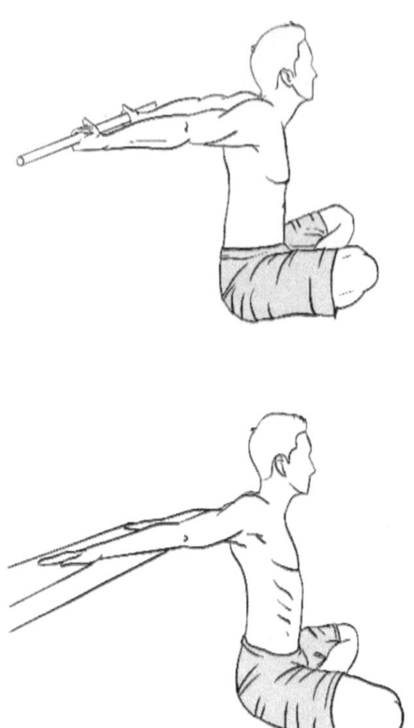

Shoulder Extension

These moves are designed to test your shoulder hyperextension.

Flexibility Test Instructions:

- Place your hands behind you, on a box or any other flat surface.
- Your palms should be flat against the surface.
- Crouch down.
- You should be able to get at least a 45-degree angle from your torso to your arm. 90 degrees if you are a gymnast or athlete, where that is needed.
- Your spine should not be rounding.

If you can do this, then you have between satisfactory and good shoulder extension flexibility. If you find this difficult, then you may have tight pecs, anterior delts, or biceps.

Mobility Test Instructions:

- Hold onto a broomstick or rod, with both hands behind you. Try this with your knuckles facing upwards (supine grip) and with your knuckles facing downward (prone grip).
- List the stick or rod upwards, with your elbows straight.
- You should get a 90-degree angle or more.

If you are unable to do this, then you may have weak rotator cuffs, posterior delts, or lats.

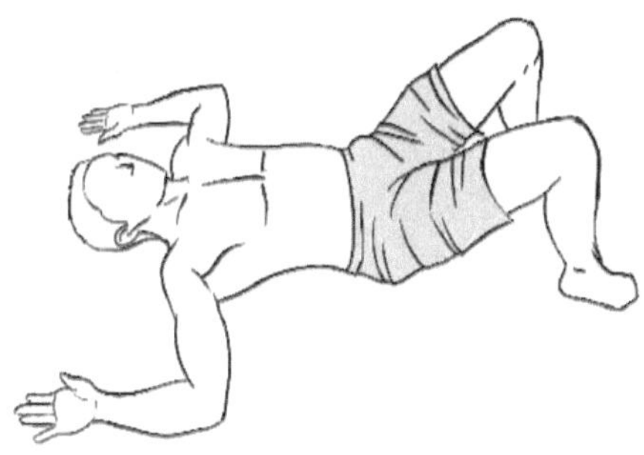

External Rotation

This move tests how well your shoulders rotate outwards.

Flexibility Test Instructions:

- Lay on the ground with your arm straight out beside you. There should be a straight line formed from your right hand all the way to your left hand.
- Bend your elbows upwards at a 90-degree angle.
- Your palms should be facing the ceiling, and the back of your hands should be flat against the floor.
- Your back should remain flat against the floor.

If you can have the backs of your hands and your back flat against the floor at the same time, then you have good external rotation. If not, then you may have tight internal rotators.

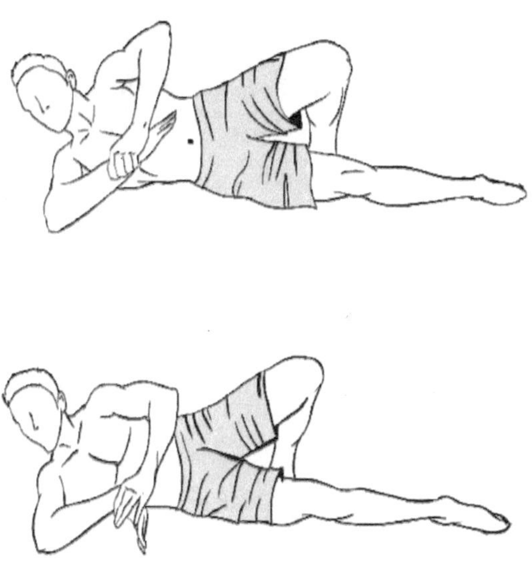

Internal Rotation

This move is designed to test how well your shoulders rotate inwards.

Flexibility Test Instructions:

- Lie down on your back. Move your body over to one side so that one side of your body is resting on the floor.
- Your arm should be about 70 degrees out from your body, with your fingers pointing to the sky.
- Pivot your arm so that your palm starts moving towards the floor, go as low as you can.
- Flex your wrist so that your fingertips touch the floor.

If you can do this, then you have good internal rotation flexibility. If you find this difficult, then it indicates that you may have tight external rotators or a tight posterior capsule.

Mobility Test Instructions:

- Place the back of your hand flat against the small of your back.
- Your scapula (shoulder blade) should be flat; it should not be sticking out.
- Move your hand up your back towards your head.
- Bring your other hand up and over your head towards the side, moving up your back.
- Try and grab the fingers of the hand, moving up the back without the scapula sticking out.

If you can do this, then your internal rotation mobility is good. If not, then you may have a weak teres major, subscapularis, serratus anterior, or lower traps.

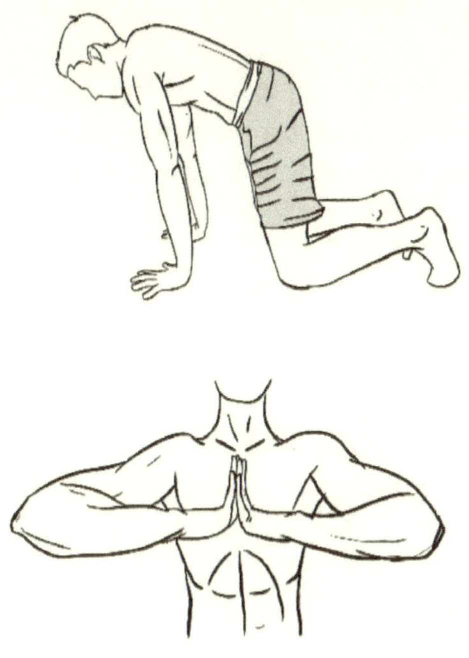

Wrist and Finger Extension

This move is designed at testing how well you can open up your wrists and fingers.

Wrist Flexibility Test Instructions:

- Get down on all fours, with your palms flat on the floor.
- Your hands should be aligned with your shoulders.
- Keep your hands straight and lean forward as far as you can.
- The palms of your hands should remain stuck to the floor at all times.

If you can do this with your arms pushing past more than 90 degrees, then you have good wrist flexibility. If not, it indicates that you have tight wrists.

Finger Extension Test Instructions:

- Place your hands together, with palms and fingers touching.
- Slowly move the bottoms of your hands apart.
- Move as far apart as you can with the entirety of your hands still touching.

If you can do this and get a 90-degree angle from the back of your hand to your fingers, then you have good finger flexibility. If not, then you will have to work on it.

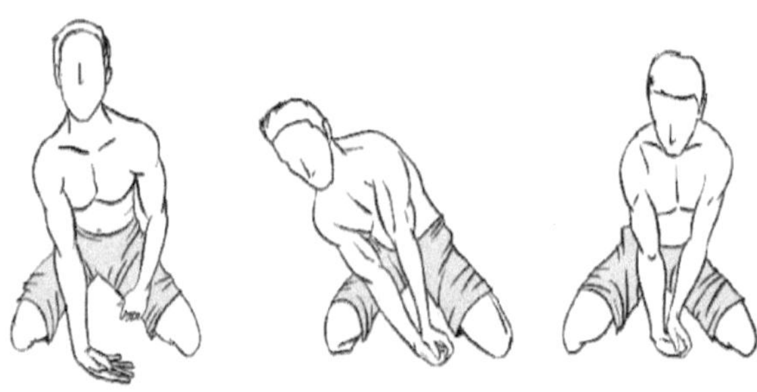

Wrist and Finger Flexion

This move tests how far your wrists and fingers move inwards.

Flexibility Test Instructions:

- Get down onto your knees, place the back of one of your hands on the floor, between your legs.
- Lean over to one side; this should be the side the arm is on. For example, if you are using your right arm, then lean over to the right.
- Roll your fingers up into a ball, so you are making a fist. The back of your hand remains on the ground.
- Slowly move your body back towards the center; your arm should stay straight.

If you can get back to the center with your arm perpendicular to the floor, then your wrist and finger flexion is at a good level. If not, then you will have to work on it.

LOWER BODY MOBILITY

The following movements and stretches will focus on the lower body and help you to identify any problem areas in that region.

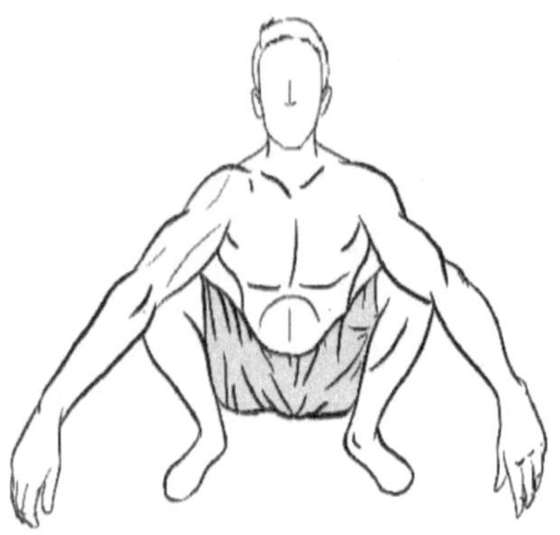

Internal Hip Rotation

This movement will test how well your hip moves inwardly. There aren't many situations where you would be doing this naturally, but it is good to have it balance out external hip rotations, which are more common.

Instructions:

- Start in a rested squat position. Go down as low as you can.
- Lean over to the right and drop the left knee in towards the floor.
- Your foot should not leave the floor. However, it is expected that it will shift over to the side.
- Touch your knee to the ground.
- Repeat on the other side.

If your knee can touch the ground, then you have good internal hip rotation.

For those that cannot get into a rested squat position, there is another move that you could try.

Instructions:

- Lay flat on your belly with your legs bent so that your legs are at a 90-degree angle.
- Let your feet drop to the sides of your body simultaneously.
- Your legs should make an angle of over 35 degrees.

If you can reach more than a 35-degree angle, then your internal hip rotation is satisfactory, but a 45-degree angle is preferable.

If you were unable to do both of these moves, then it indicates that you have tight external rotators or tight glutes.

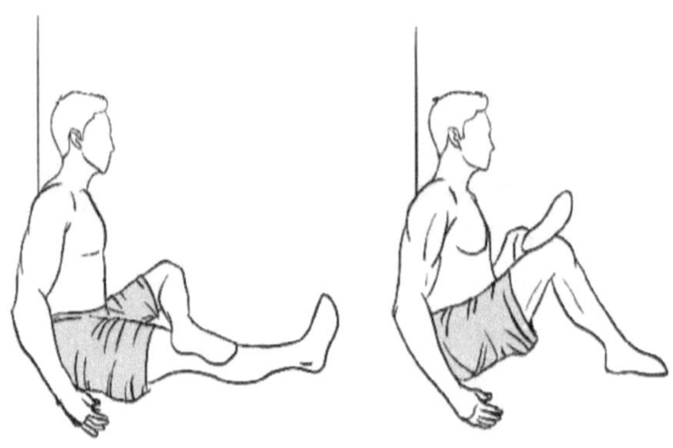

External Hip Rotation and Hip Flexion

This will test how well your hips can move and rotate outwardly.

Instructions:

- Sit up straight with your back flat against a wall.
- Stretch your legs out straight in front of you and bring your left leg over your right knee. Your left ankle should be touching the right knee.
- Bring your right knee up as high as you can go.
- You may repeat on the other side if desired, to see if you get different results.

If you can get your left leg (in this case) up to your chest, then you have really good flexibility. However, about 45 degrees away from your chest is satisfactory. If you are unable to get this close, then you probably have a tight TFL (tensor fascia lata; part of your hip muscles), piriformis, or glutes.

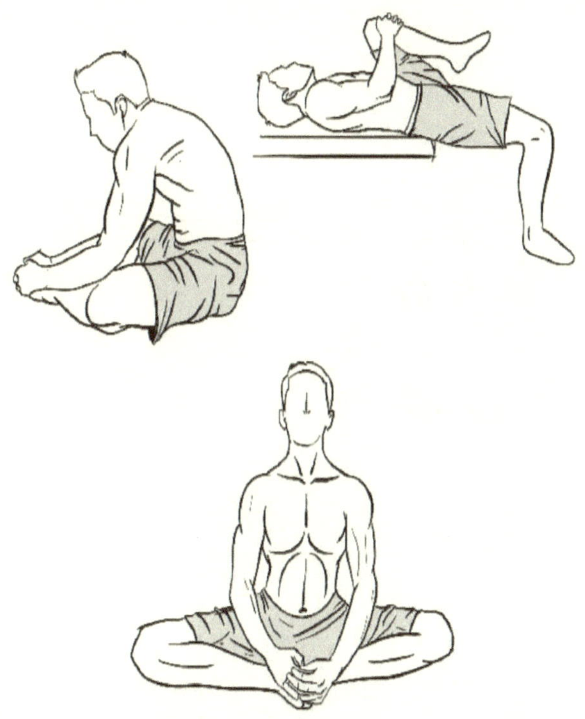

Hip Abduction and External Hip Rotation

This move will test how far your leg can move away from your midline, think of doing a side-kick or leg lift.

Instructions:

- Start by sitting on the floor on your sit bones; your back should be straight. Make sure you are not on your tailbone.
- Bring your feet together, so the bottoms are touching.
- Pull your feet into your body and try and push down your knees to

touch the floor.

If your feet are brought in as much as they can go, and you can get your knees to touch the ground, you are pretty flexible. If not, then you probably have tight adductors and internal rotators.

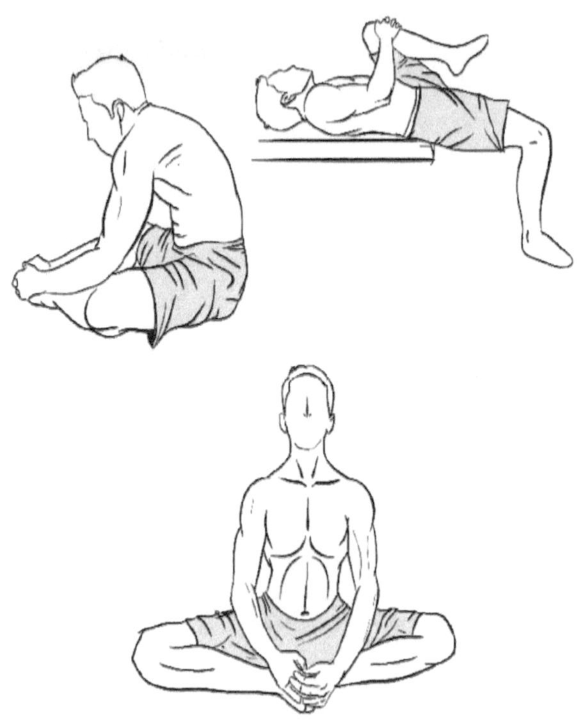

Hip Extension

A good hip extension will allow your leg to move behind you.

Instructions:

- Lie down on your back, on a hard flat surface. The best place would be a table or a bench.
- Your whole back should be on the surface with your butt half on and

half off.

- Bring your right knee up to your chest, bring it in as close as you can and push your back into the surface.
- Allow your left leg to hang off the edge of the surface. Your knee should be bent at a 90-degree angle.
- Your leg should hang past the edge of the surface, at an angle over 180 degrees. Your back should never leave the surface.

If your leg hangs over the surface and is not pulled upwards, then you have a good hip extension. If you are unable to do this, then you probably have tight hip flexors or tight quads. If you notice that your leg moves outwards, then you probably have weak adductors or a tight TFL.

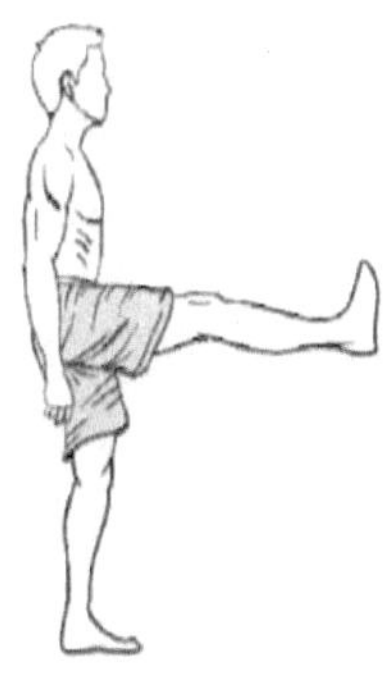

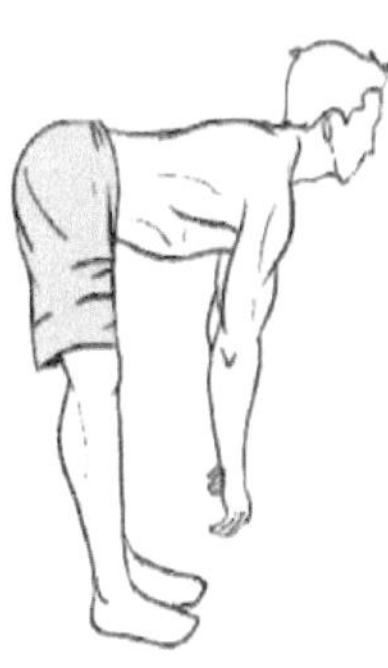

Pike

The pike position is just a forward bend, but you can feel it in the muscles of your leg.

Pike Flexibility Test Instructions:

- Start by standing up straight with your feet together.
- Bend over at your hips, keeping your back straight.
- Keep your knees locked.
- Try and get down as low as possible with your back still straight.

If you can get your back to lay 90 degrees from your legs, then you have satisfactory pike flexibility. For those more flexible, you can try and touch your palms to the ground about two feet from your legs. If you are unable to get a minimum of the 90-degree angle, this indicates that you have tight hamstrings, calves, and Achilles tendons.

Pike Mobility Test Instructions:

- Start by standing up straight.
- Kick one of your legs out in front of you without bending either knee or your back.
- Try and get your leg up to a 90-degree angle, right out in front of you.

If you are unable to get your leg up to 90 degrees, then this indicates that you may have weak hip flexors and a weak rectus femoris.

Ankle Dorsiflexion

This movement tests the mobility of your ankle. It is important to have strong ankles as they are part of what holds us up and helps us to keep moving.

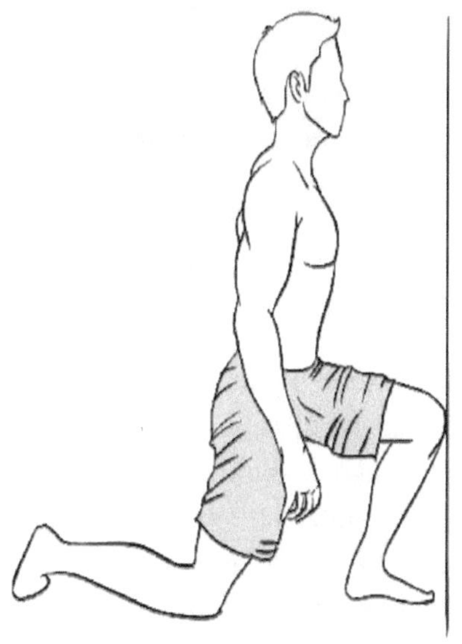

Instructions:

- Start by getting into a lunge position by a wall. Your knee and toe of one leg should be touching the wall, while the other leg is out behind you.
- Place a ruler underneath your foot or right beside it.
- Move your foot backward an inch at a time. Your knee should remain fixed to the wall.
- Once you have reached five inches, you may stop. Make sure the heel of your foot never lifts off the ground.

If you can reach the five inches away from the wall, this shows that your dorsiflexion is good. If not, then this is an indicator that you may have a tight soleus or Achilles tendon.

If you are finding yourself having a mobility or flexibility problem with a muscle you didn't even know existed, you do not need to worry. As long as you know, it is in your back or hip or wherever, that is okay. I am going to provide you with stretches to cover all areas that will certainly target that obscure muscle you haven't heard of and improve that problem area.

CONCLUDING THOUGHTS ON THE MOBILITY AND FLEXIBILITY TEST

Once you have completed the mobility and flexibility test, you should have a good idea of where your problem areas lie. I know this seems like a lot, but I am confident this will not take you long and will provide you with an excellent gauge of where you are right now. Do not feel discouraged if you are unable to do some or even all of the moves; that is why I wrote this book. I want to help you along your journey of regaining flexibility and mobility.

In order to move forward, you needed to know where you are right now. Now that you are entirely aware of what you are capable of and what you need to improve on, we can begin giving you the tools you need to succeed at your goal of increased mobility and flexibility.

2

CONDITIONING: ALL THE STRETCHES YOU WILL EVER NEED TO KNOW

The stretches that are mentioned in this chapter will be focused on resolving short term problems. Sometimes we sit or sleep funny, and that causes our muscles and joints to hurt. I'm sure you have woken up with a stiff neck from sleeping in an uncomfortable position. This sort of thing is very common and doesn't usually have any long term damage, but it does cause discomfort. When you are uncomfortable or sore, you will not perform at your best. Stretches are the best way to get rid of that pain and discomfort so you can get back to feeling your best.

The stretches below are broken up into body part specific stretches. This will help you navigate the chapter easier, and if you have a specific problem, you know where to find the solution. Let's get into the stretches.

NECK, SHOULDER, AND CHEST

Many people suffer from some sort of tightness or discomfort in these areas. This is usually due to the way we sit at our computers or the way we sleep. Whatever the cause, it can be very uncomfortable to deal with. The following stretches will help relieve tension, stiffness, and discomfort from the chest, neck, and shoulders.

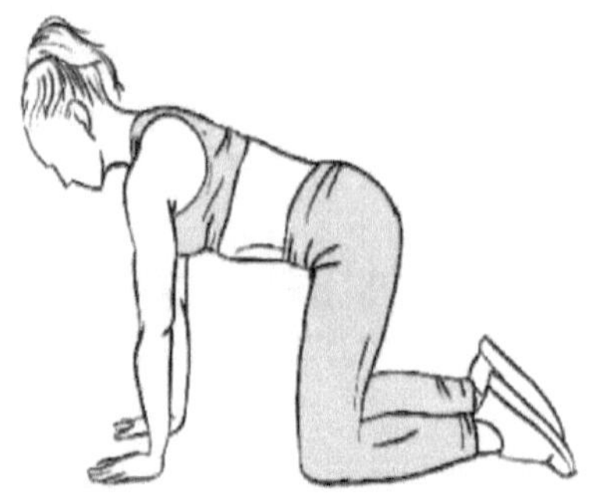

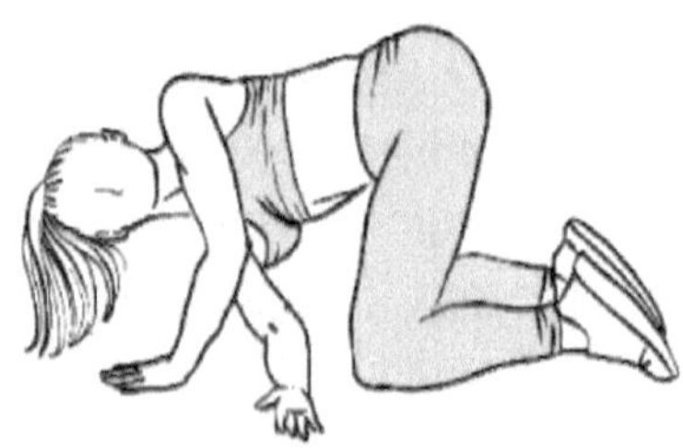

Thread the Needle

This stretch targets your shoulder girdle muscles and a muscle in your chest called the pectoralis minor.

Instructions:

- Begin by kneeling down on all fours; your hands should be aligned with your shoulders and your knees with your hips.
- Take your right arm and stretch it through the space between your left arm and thigh. Your palm should be facing up.
- Bend your left arm to allow the right side of your body to have more movement. You should be able to feel it at the back of the right shoulder.
- Hold for a couple of seconds, repeat a few more times before moving

on to the other side.

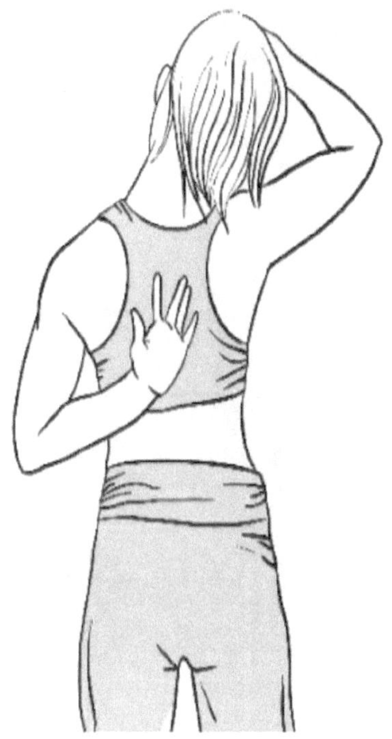

Upper Trapezius Stretch

This stretch will target your neck muscles; it gives the muscles a nice long stretch.

Instructions:

- Begin by sitting or standing with your back straight.
- Place one hand on your back; it can be on your lower back or between your shoulder blades.
- Take the other hand, place it to the opposite side of your head and pull your head to your shoulder.

- You should feel a stretch in your neck on the opposite side of the arm, pulling your head down. Hold for 20 to 30 seconds and then repeat on the other side.

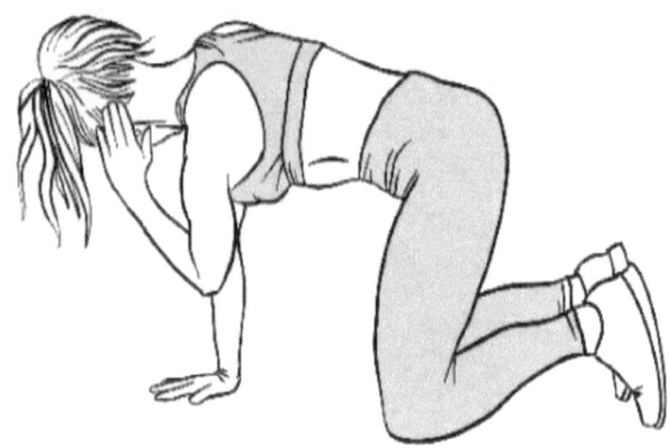

Quadruped Thoracic Rotation Stretch

This stretch targets the upper part of your spine.

Instructions:

- Begin on all fours. Align your hands with your shoulders and your knees with your hips. Your core should be engaged, and your back should remain straight at all times.
- Touch the back of your head with your right hand, do not put pressure on your head.

- Slowly move your head and shoulder inward towards your opposite arm.
- Then move all the way back, past the starting point until your elbow points up to the ceiling.
- Return to the middle position after holding for a couple of seconds.
- Do this for about 30 seconds then repeat on the other side.

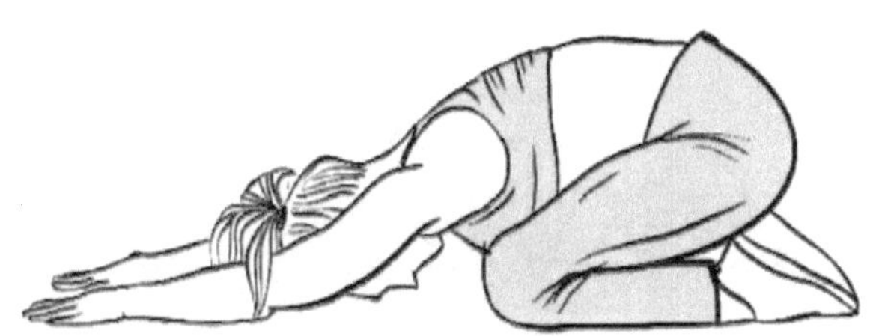

Child's Pose

This is a simple yoga move that helps with your neck, back, and shoulders. You should also feel it in your glutes and hips.

Instructions:

- Kneel on the floor and sit on your heels. Your knees should be a bit wider than your hips, and your feet should be touching.

- Fold your body over so that your torso is lying on your thighs. Reach your arms out in front of you so that they are over your head. Place your forehead on the ground.
- Pull your chest and shoulders towards the floor; this will cause a deeper stretch.
- Hold this position for 30 seconds before repeating.

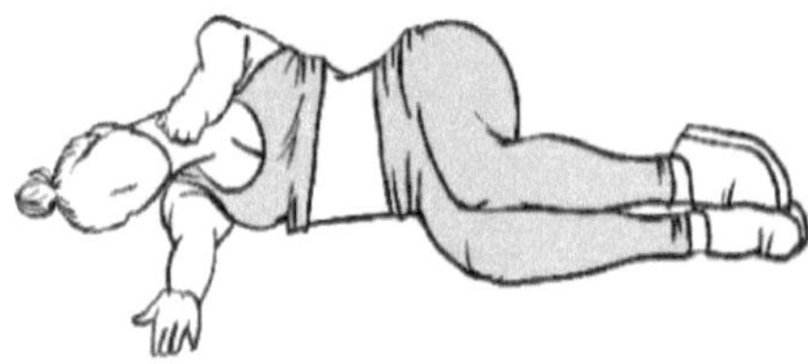

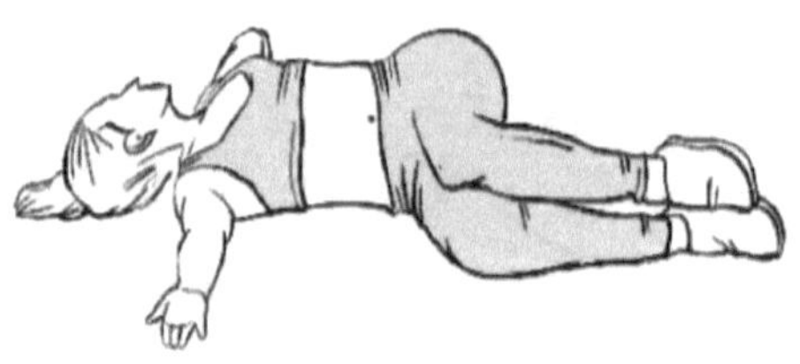

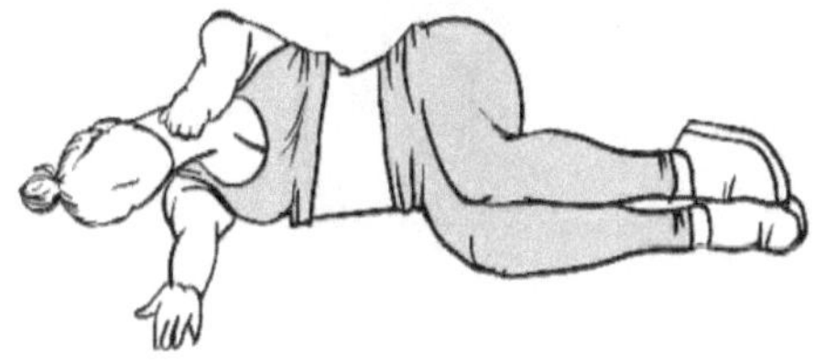

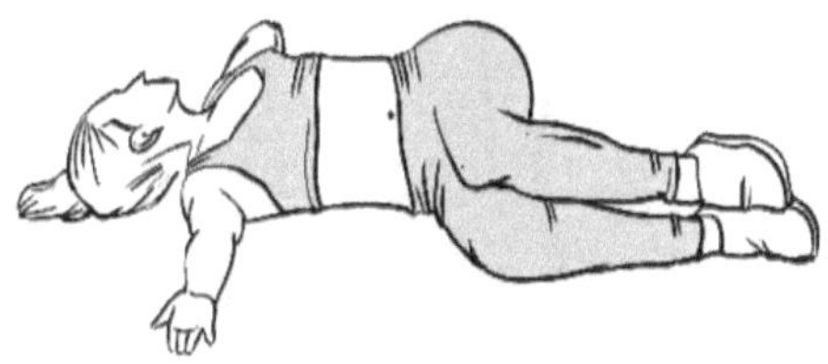

T-spine Windmill Stretch

This stretch targets many muscles in your shoulder.

Instructions:

- Lie down on your side with your arms stretched out in front of you, your knees and hips bent at a 90-degree angle.
- Lay your arms on top of each other and the same with your legs.
- Move your top hand over to the other side of your body; you should now be laying with both arms stretched out on opposite sides to form a T shape.
- Slowly return to the starting position.
- Repeat about 5 to 10 times before repeating on the other side.

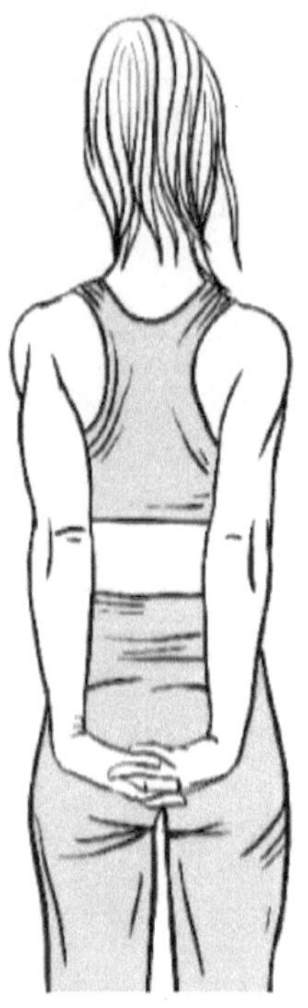

Reverse Shoulder Stretch

This stretch will target your deltoids and the pecs.

Instructions:

- Start by interlocking your fingers behind your back with your palms facing up.
- Your back and arms should be straight, and you should be pulling your shoulder blades together.
- Push your arms upward so that you can feel a stretch in your pec muscles.
- Hold this pose for about 30 seconds.

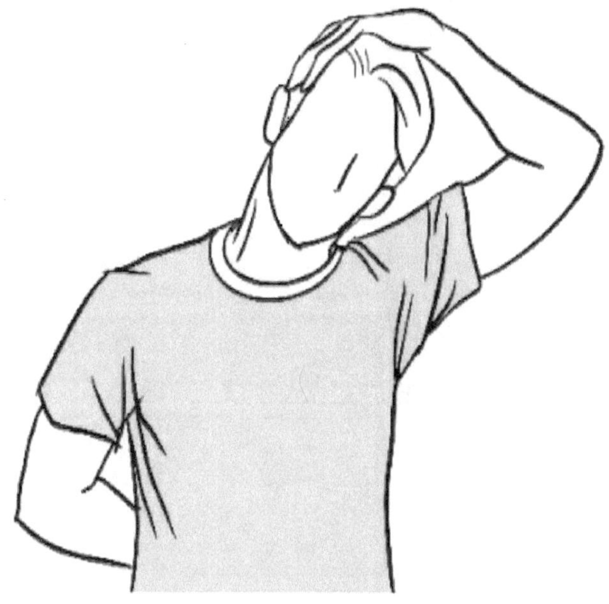

Cervical Side Bend

This stretch will help relieve the tension in the neck muscles.

Instructions:

- Sit or Stand with your back and neck straight.
- Move your right ear to your right shoulder, while you keep looking straight in front of you.
- You should feel the stretch in your left neck muscles. Hold for a few seconds and then repeat on the other side.

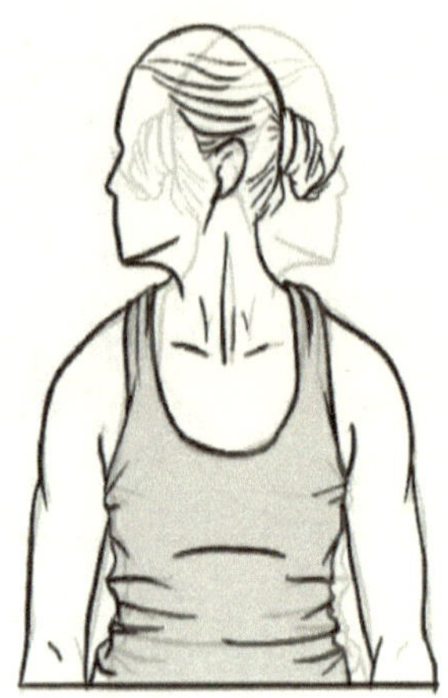

Cervical Rotation

This stretch also focuses specifically on the neck muscles.

Instructions:

- Turn your head to one side; make sure not to move your shoulders.
- Hold for a few seconds then turn to the other side.
- If you would like to add some pressure use your hand push against your chin gently.

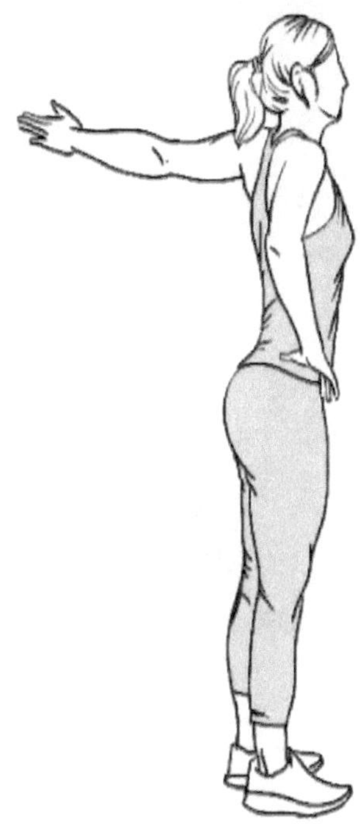

Wall Chest Stretch

This movement will allow you to stretch out your chest muscles.

Instructions:

- Place a straight arm on a wall.
- Take a step forward with the leg furthest away from the wall.
- Gently move your chest forward and feel the stretch in your chest.
- You may move your hand lower or higher on the wall to stretch out the various sections in your chest.
- Repeat the process on the other side

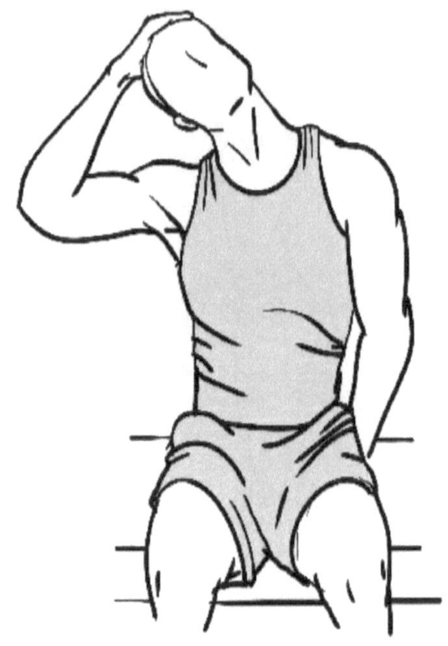

Anterior Scalene Stretch

Sometimes neck stiffness is caused by the anterior scalene muscle; this stretch will target that muscle.

Instructions:

- Place your right hand on your head.
- Start slowly pulling your head to the side so that your right ear moves closer to your right shoulder.
- Hold this pose for about 30 seconds and repeat three times before moving on to the other side.

ARMS, HANDS, AND WRISTS

When it comes to stretching, we often forget about our wrists, hands, and arms. However, these are important parts of our body and should not be neglected. If you are someone who is typing for most of the day, having any kind of discomfort or stiffness in these areas can really slow you down. There are a few stretches that can ease that feeling and help you get your mobility back.

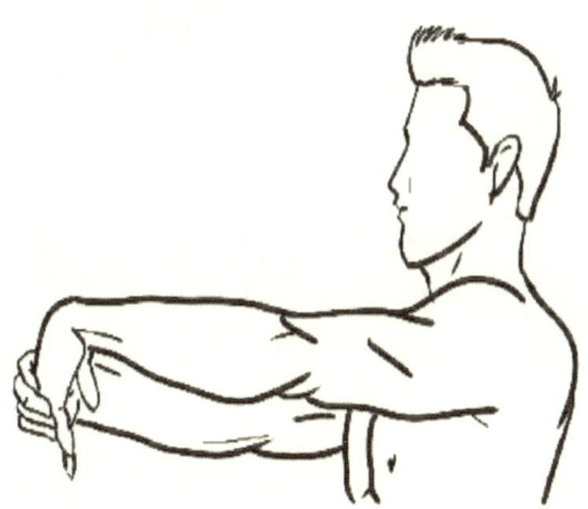

Wrist Extensor Stretch

This is a popular stretch to relieve tightness in your wrists.

Instructions:

- Lift your hand out in front of you and bend your wrist down so your palm faces you.

- Use your other hand to pull your bent wrist further towards you gently. You should feel the stretch in your forearm and wrist.
- Hold for 30 seconds and repeat three times. Repeat on the other hand.

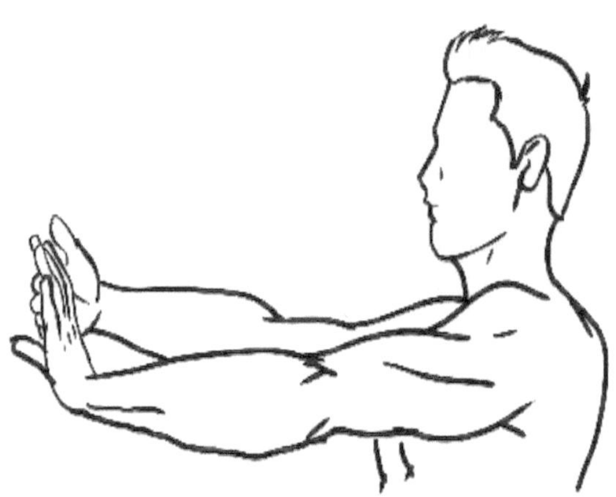

Wrist Flexor Stretch

This stretch is just the opposite of the previous stretch. It stretches the muscles on the inside of your wrist and arm.

Instructions:

- Stretch your hand out in front of you with your palm facing down.
- Bend your wrist upwards.
- Take the other and gently pull your wrist back towards you until you feel the stretch down your forearm.

- Hold for 30 seconds and repeat three times. Repeat on the other hand.

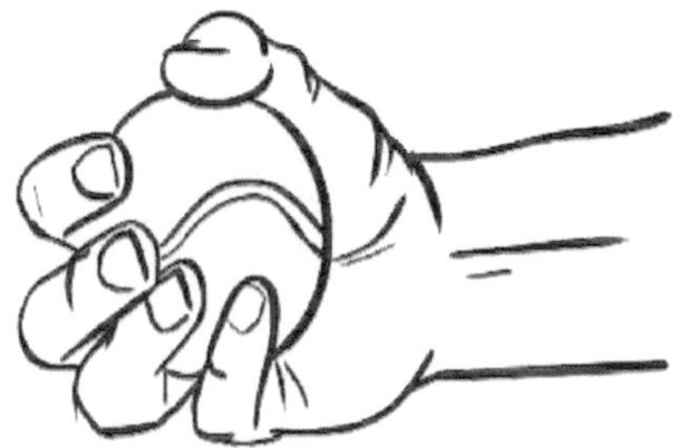

Tennis Ball Squeeze

This stretch targets the muscles and joints in the hand and wrist.

Instructions:

- Hold a tennis ball in one hand and squeeze it as hard as you can.
- Hold this for about 4 or 5 seconds then slowly release.
- Repeat this fifteen times before moving onto the other hand

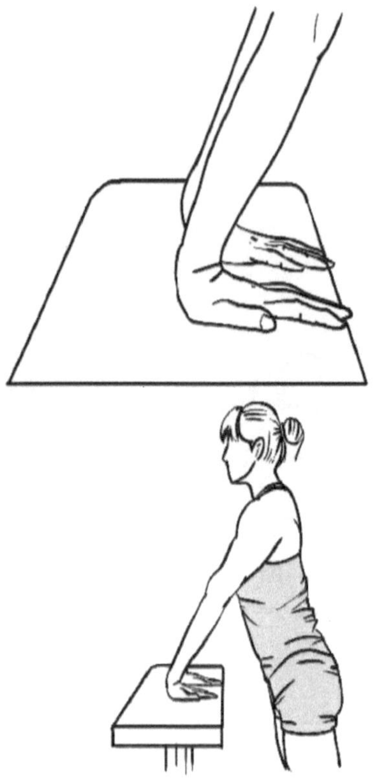

Desk Press

This stretch targets your wrists and forearms.

Instructions:

- Find a desk or table, place your hands on the surface with your wrists turned, so your fingers are pointing at you.
- Gently push forward until you feel the stretch in your forearm.
- Hold for 15 seconds, repeat this about ten times.

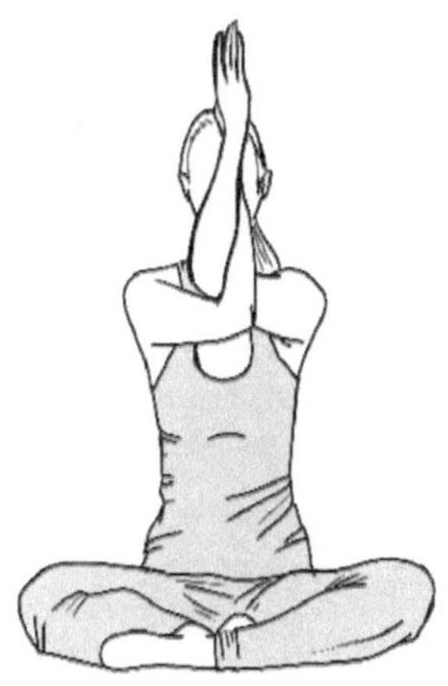

Eagle Arms

This stretch is excellent for stretching out your wrists and shoulders.

Instructions:

- Sit or stand up straight with your arms in front of you.
- Cross your left and right arms, with the right arm on top.
- Move both elbows, so they are bent upwards.
- Intertwine your arms so that the palms of both hands are touching.
- Move both arms away from your body in an upward motion; you should feel a spread between your shoulder blades.
- Stay in this pose for five deep breaths, then switch hands.

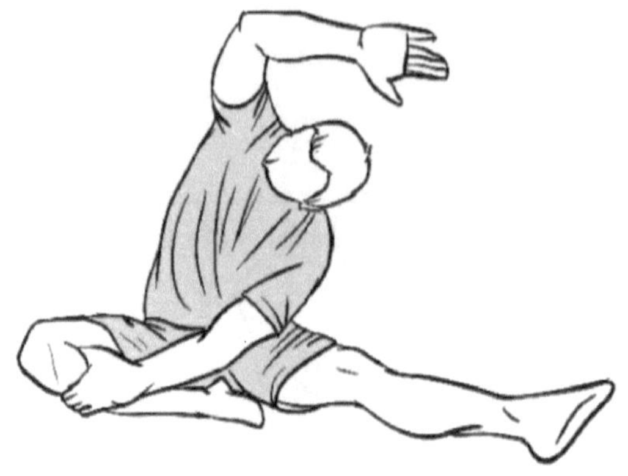

Assisted Side Bend

This move stretches out your arms but also lengthens your torso.

Instructions:

- Sit with your back straight.
- Move your arms so that they are above your head.
- Grab the wrist of one hand with the other and pull yourself over to the side.
- If you feel your ribs flaring, shift them back so that the stretch is only felt through your side and arm.
- Hold this for 30 seconds or until you feel ready, then switch over to the other side.

BACK AND TORSO

Suffering from a tight back can restrict your range of movement. The following stretches will allow you to gain back the mobility in your back.

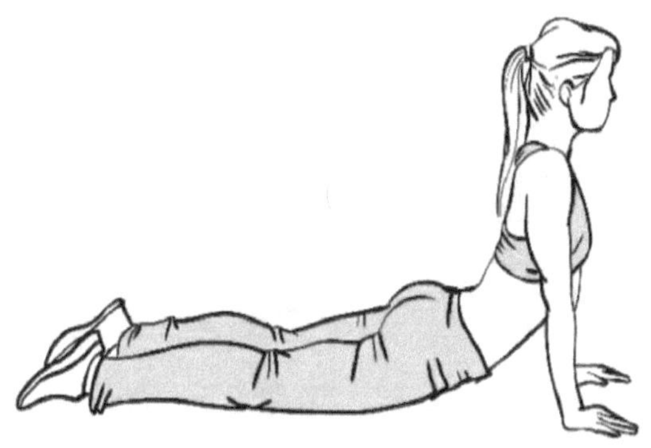

The Cobra

This stretch lengthens the whole upper body and is ideal if you suffer from pain related to sitting uncomfortably at a desk.

Instructions:

- Lay down with your belly to the floor.
- Bring your hands directly under your shoulders, breathe in and push up with your hands.

- Once your arms are completely straight, look up to the ceiling to stretch out your neck. Hold for about 30 seconds.
- Slowly exhale and bring yourself back down.
- Repeat this about three times.

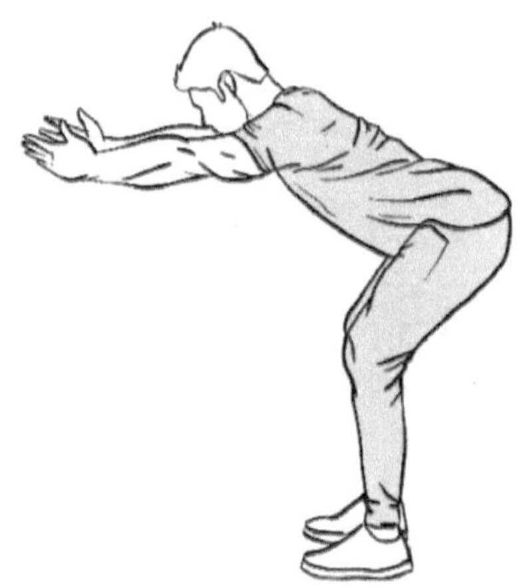

Hip Hinge

This stretch is especially useful for your lower back.

Instructions:

- Stand up with your back straight and your feet apart. You should be a few feet away from the wall.
- Leave your hands hanging to your side or out in front of you. Then bend your knees slightly, and bend at your pelvis, so your whole torso moves towards the ground.

- Once your back is parallel to the ground, slowly bring yourself back
  up to the starting position.

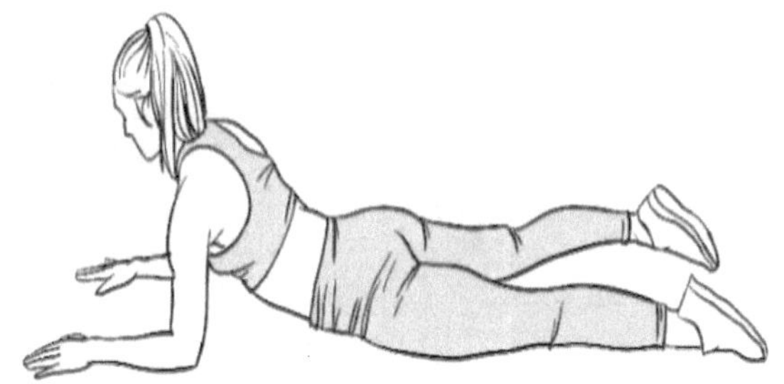

Sphinx Pose

This pose is common in yoga and is used to strengthen the spine and stretch
out the abdomen.

Instructions:

- Begin by laying on your belly, the tops of your feet should be facing
  down.
- Bring your arms in and lift yourself up so your elbows and shoulders
  are in line. Your palms should be flat on the ground, and your

forearms should be parallel to each other.

- Inhale and push down on your forearms and lift your head and chest towards the ceiling.
- Engage your core and glutes, push your pelvis into the ground.
- Hold this pose for ten breaths and then relax and bring yourself back down slowly.

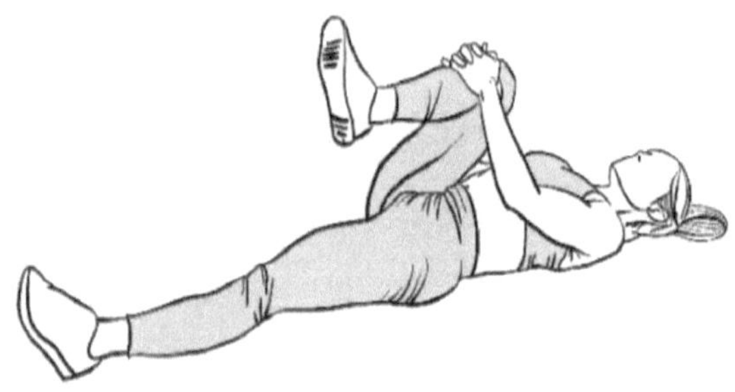

Knee-to-chest stretch

This stretch really targets the lower back.

Instructions:

- Lay flat on your back and bring your right knee up to your chest.

- With both hands, grab the shin of your right leg and pull it down so that you drive the leg into your chest. If this is too tricky, bend your left leg.
- Do not lift your hips, really try and lengthen your spine.
- Hold this pose for 5 to 30 seconds, release and then repeat at least three times before moving to the other leg.

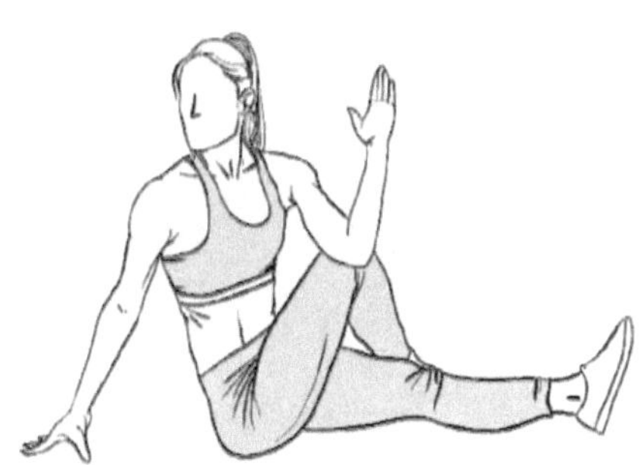

Piriformis stretch

This stretch will help release any tension in your buttocks, lower back, and hips.

Instructions:

- Lay down on your back and have your knees bent.
- Take your right ankle and place it over your left thigh.

- Grab your left thigh and pull it towards your chest, get as close to your chest as you can.
- Hold this pose for 30 to 60 seconds, then repeat on the other leg.

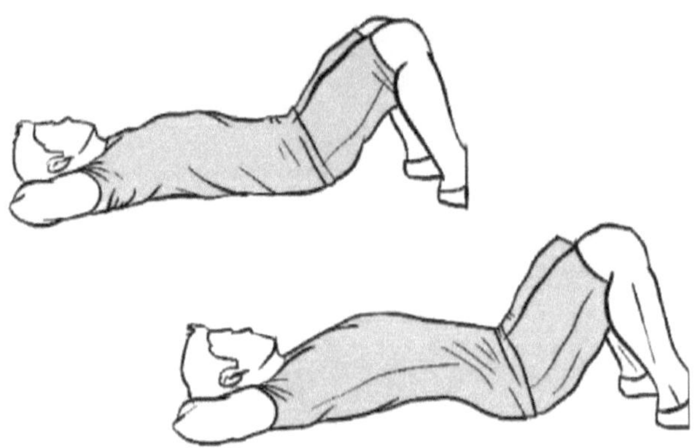

Pelvic tilt

This stretch can relieve pain and stiffness in your lower back and strengthen your abdomen.

Instructions:

- Lay on your back on the floor and your knees bent. Your hands should be to your side with palms flat on the floor.
- Flatten your back to the floor and engage your core muscles.
- Hold for 5 to 10 seconds and then slowly release. Repeat as many times as desired.

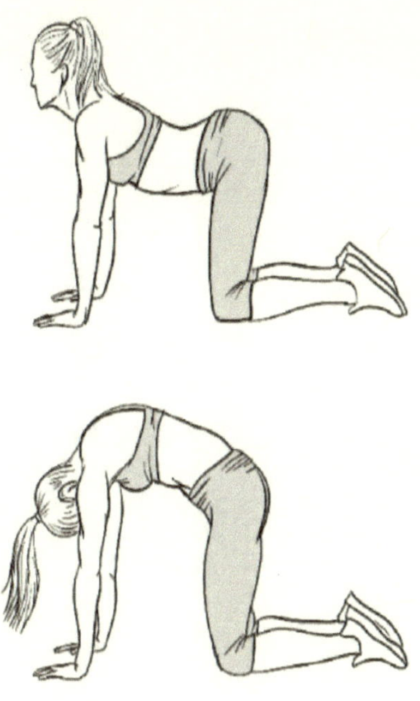

Cat-cow stretch

This move stretches out your spine and your upper body.

Instructions:

- Start on all fours.
- Breathe in, push your belly towards the ground, and lift your head.
- Then in one smooth movement exhale, tuck your chin in and lift your spine to the ceiling.
- Do this repeatedly for about 60 seconds.

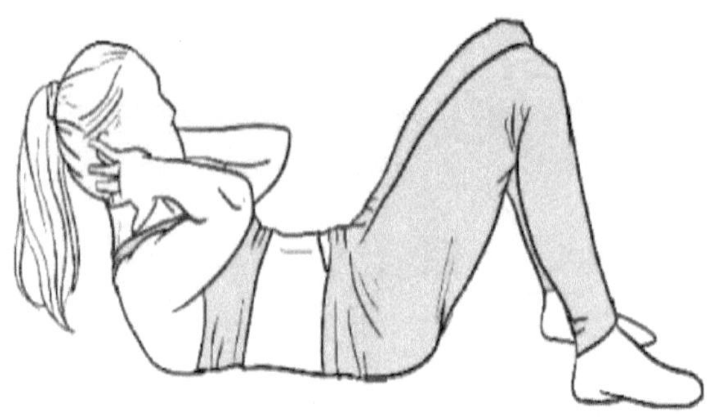

Partial Crunch

This move can stabilize your spine if you suffer or are recovering from back pain.

Instructions:

- Lay down on your back with your knees bent and feet on the floor.
- Push your lower back into the floor and engage your core.
- Lift your head and shoulders slightly off the ground by reaching for your feet with your hands. Use your core muscles, not your neck, to support this movement.

- Hold this for 1 to 3 minutes. Then relax and repeat.

HIPS AND GLUTES

Tight hips are something many people struggle with; sometimes, you will feel it when you sit. Your glutes are the biggest muscle in your body, so it is essential to pay attention to it, both of these areas work together when it comes to mobility and flexibility.

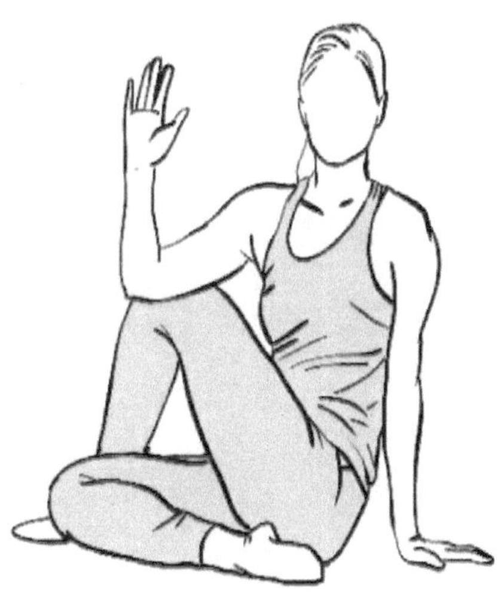

Half Lord of the Fishes

This stretch targets your spine and hips.

Instructions:

- Start by sitting on the floor, swing your left foot over your right thigh. Bend your right leg so your foot is as close to your butt as you can get it.
- Place your right elbow on the outside of your left knee and place your left hand just behind you for support.
- Keep your left foot firmly on the ground as you stretch.
- Hold for at least 30 seconds then repeat on the other side.

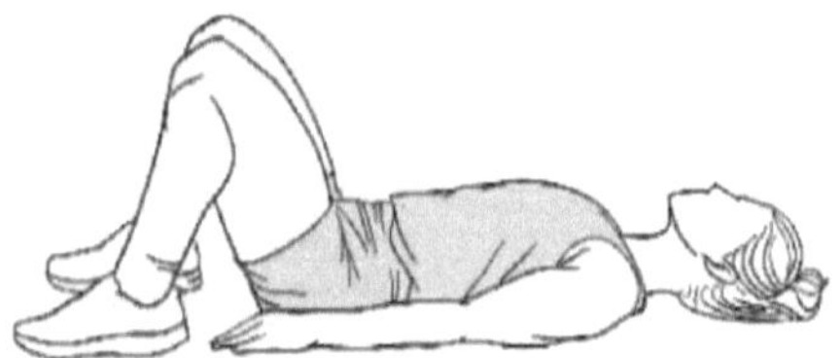

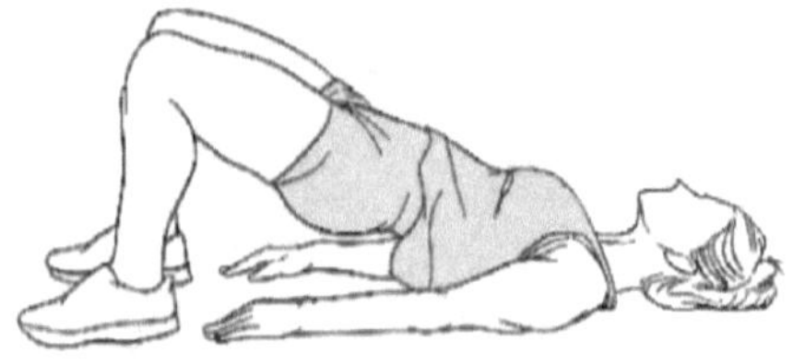

Glute Bridge

This exercise activates the glutes and works via a hip extension.

Instructions:

- Lay on your back, with your knees bent and feet hip-width apart.

- Lift your pelvis towards the ceiling by engaging your glutes and driving your heels into the ground.
- Hold for 5 to 10 seconds, then slowly bring yourself back down again. Repeat ten to fifteen times.

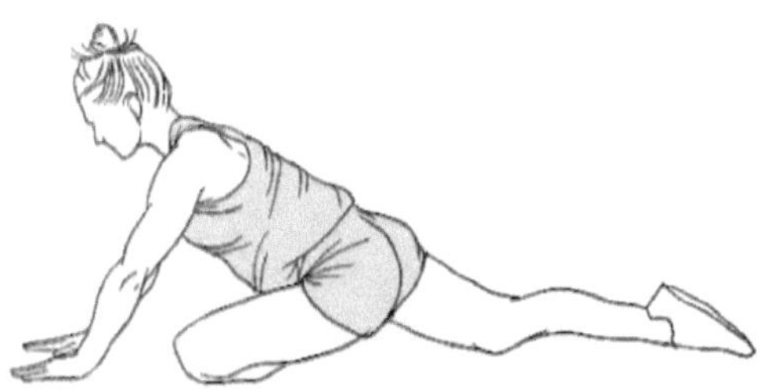

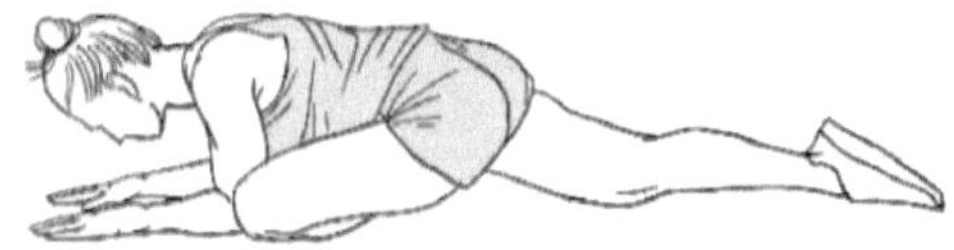

Pigeon Pose

This is an excellent stretch for those on their feet a lot as it stretches the glutes, hips, and piriformis.

Instructions:

- Start by getting down on your right knee. Drop your left knee to the left and slide your right leg behind you.
- Push your hips into the ground and walk your hands forward on the

ground as far as you can. Palms should be facing the ground.
- Keep your hips centered.
- Hold this pose for 20 to 30 seconds. Repeat on the other side.

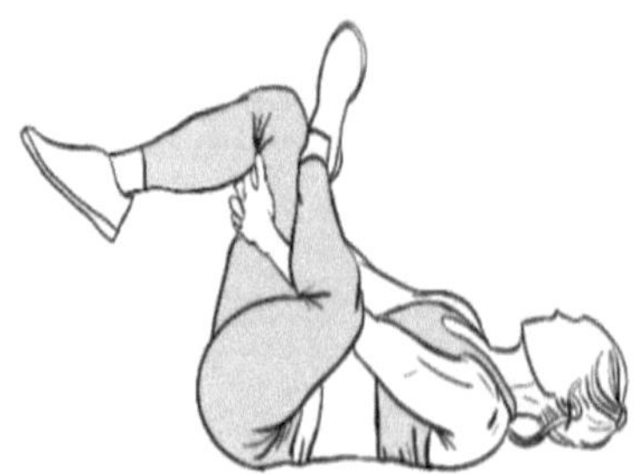

Lying Figure 4 Stretch

This move gives a great stretch to your glutes and hip flexors.

Instructions:

- Lay down on your back with your legs bent and feet off the ground.
- Place your right ankle over your left thigh.
- Grab your left thigh and pull both legs toward your chest.

- Hold for at least 20 seconds. Repeat on the other side.

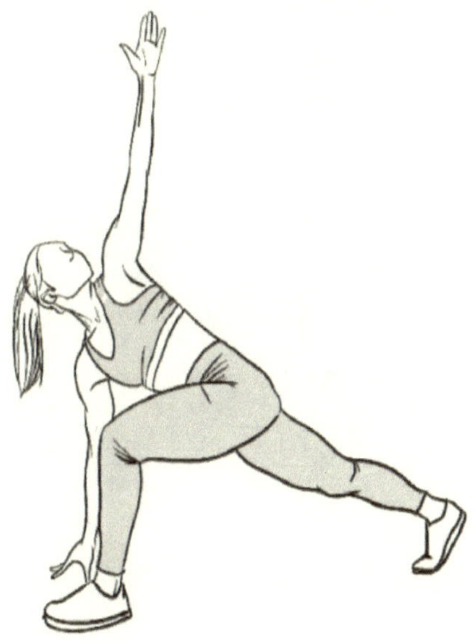

Lunge with Spinal Twist

This move will stretch out the hip flexors, back, and quads

Instructions:

- Stand up straight with your feet together, then take a large step
  forward with your right leg.
- Then drop your right knee, so you are in a lunge position. The back
  leg should be stretched out behind you.
- Put your left hand on the floor for stability and reach up to the ceiling
  with your right hand; this should cause your upper body to twist.
  Look up at your right hand.

- Hold for at least 30 seconds. Repeat with the left side.

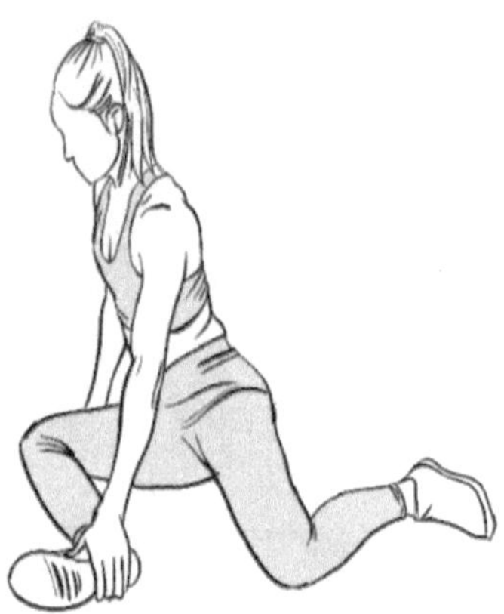

90/90 Stretch

This stretch is designed to stretch out the tightness in the hips.

Instructions:

- Sit on the floor with your left leg out in front of you, bend it at a 90-degree angle. It should be flat on the ground with your foot flexed and facing the right.
- Move your right knee to the left of you and bend your knee and flex the foot; it should be facing behind you.
- Your left butt cheek should be on the ground, now try and get your right butt cheek as close to the ground as possible by pushing your

hips downwards.

- Hold for at least 30 seconds and repeat on the other side.

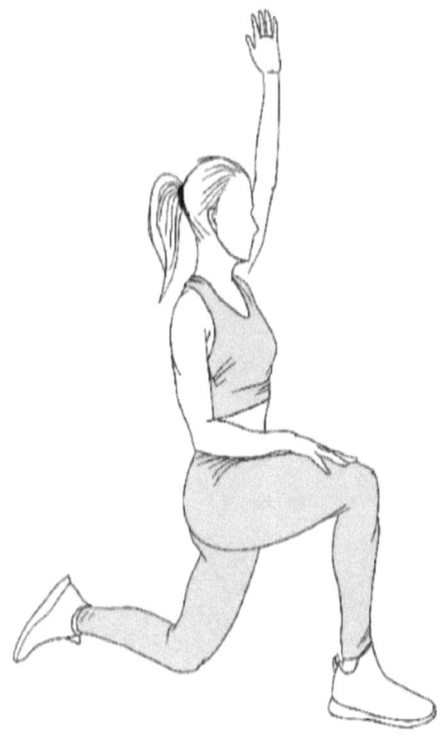

Lunging Hip Flexor Stretch

This stretch opens up the hips.

Instructions:

- Get down on one knee. One foot should be in front of you at a 90-degree angle, and the other should be bent behind you, the top of the foot flat on the ground.
- Lean forward as you try and push your hips towards the floor.
- Squeeze your butt and lift the arm on the opposite side of your front

leg.

- Hold for 30 seconds and then repeat on the other side.

Knees and Thighs

Knee pain can really get in the way of our everyday lives. If there is tightness in our thighs, that might also contribute to pain in the knees. The following stretches will help with discomfort in your knee and thigh areas.

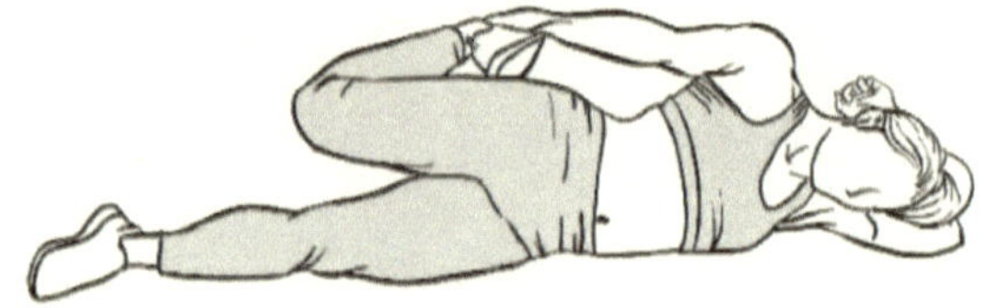

Quad Stretch

This stretch is designed to ease tension in the quads that might also be felt in the knee area.

Instructions:

- Lay down on your side with your legs stacked on top of each other. Use the arm closest to the ground to hold you up.
- Bend your top leg at the knee and grab your foot with your free hand.
- Pull the foot towards your butt until you feel the stretch in your quad.
- Hold this position for at least 30 seconds then repeat on the other side.

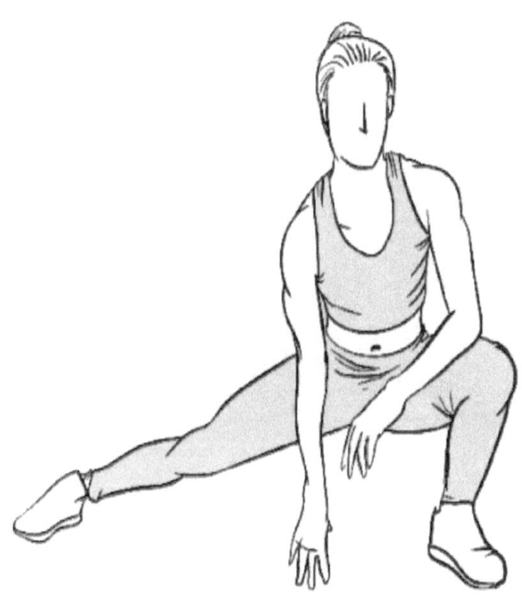

Side Lunge

This stretch targets your adductors (inner thigh muscles).

Instructions:

- Get into the side lunge position by stretching out one of your legs to the side and bending the other knee.
- Keep as much of the foot of the stretched leg on the floor as you can.

- You may place your fingertips on the ground if you need extra stability.
- Get as low as you can and hold for 15 to 30 seconds then repeat on the other side.

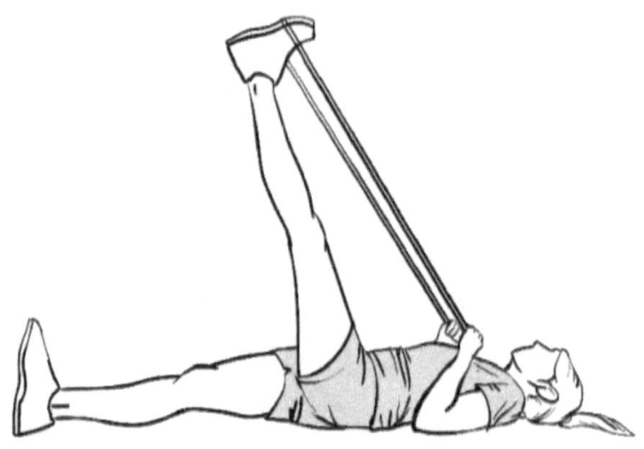

Supine Hamstring Stretch

This stretch is especially good for your hamstrings in your thighs.

Instructions:

- Lie down on your back with your knees bent.
- Use a towel or resistance bands to wrap around on your thigh and pull it towards you. The other leg can be bent, or you can straighten it out for more of a stretch.

- Try and keep the leg that you are pulling as straight as possible.
- Hold it as close to your body as possible for 30 to 60 seconds. Repeat three times, then switch to the other side.

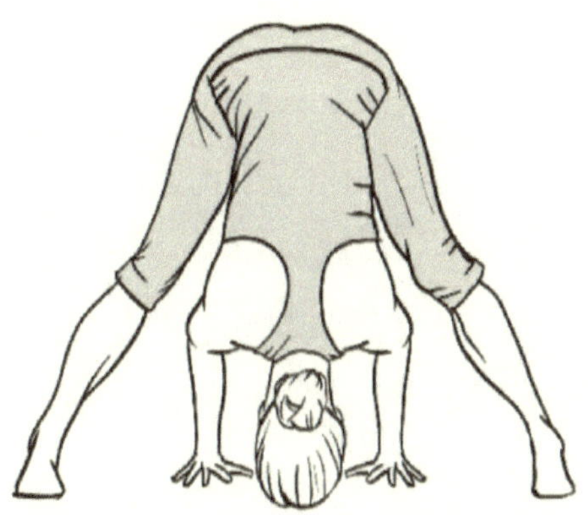

Wide-Legged Forward Fold

This stretch will target those thigh muscles.

Instructions:

- Stand with your legs 3 to 4 feet apart, could be wider depending on your height.
- Stand up straight and plant your feet into the ground, your feet should be parallel not facing inward.
- Breathe in, and as you exhale, bend at the hips, keeping your back

nice and straight.
- Try and reach for the ground with your fingers, getting your head as close to the ground as possible.
- Hold this position for at least five breaths.

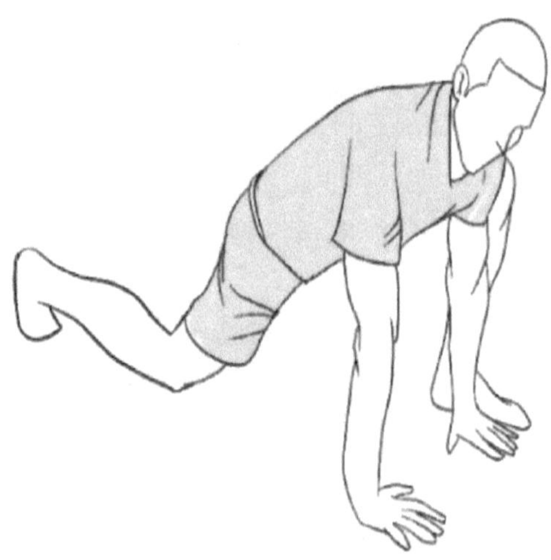

The Knight Stretch

This stretch is designed to stretch out your thighs and open up your hips.

Instructions:

- Get into the lunge position, with one leg bent down behind you and one bent up in front of you.
- Breathe in, push your chest outwards, and lean forward with your hips. Stretch it out as far as you can.

- Hold for 30 seconds and repeat five times on each side.

LOWER LEG, ANKLES, AND FEET

These parts of our body are the base of your body, and they need to be strong. Tight ankles can cause pain when walking, so it is important to get mobility back in these areas.

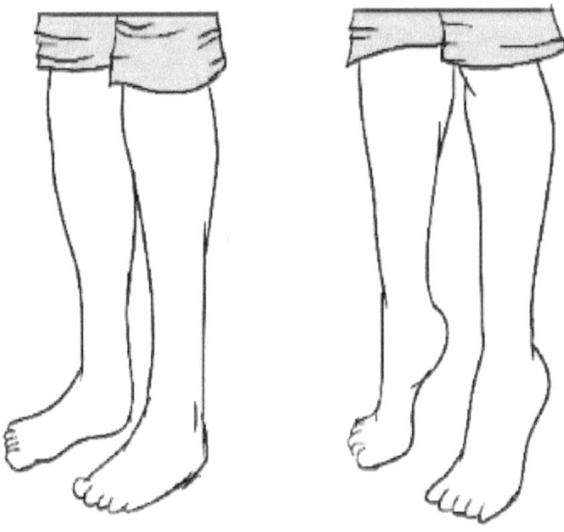

Tip Toe Tense

This stretch will stretch out the whole lower leg area.

Instructions:

- Stand up straight, then lift yourself onto your tiptoes.
- Hold for about 5 seconds, then bring yourself back down slowly and controlled.
- Repeat about ten to fifteen times.

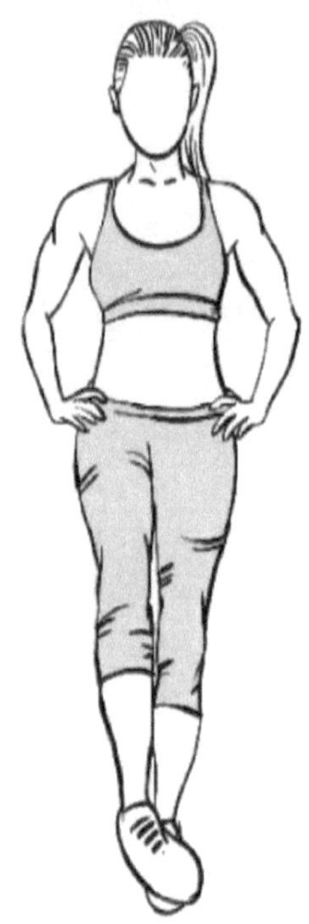

Ankle Rotation

This move will help with ankle stiffness.

Instructions:

- You may be lying down or sitting for this move.
- Lift your foot off the ground and rotate your ankle to the left, hold for a few seconds.
- Then rotate your ankle to the right, hold for a few seconds.

- You may do this as many times as desired. Repeat on the other foot.

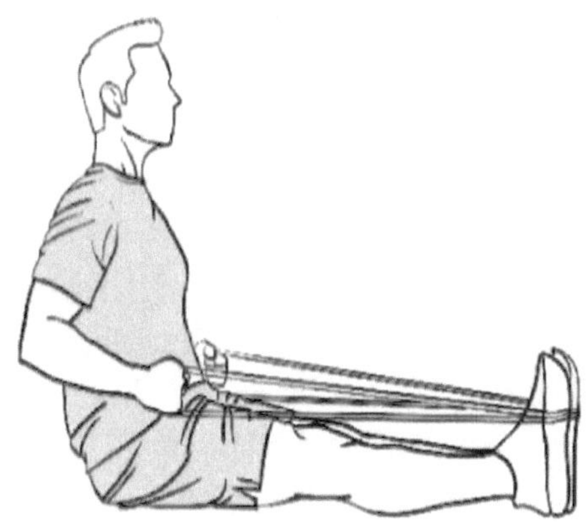

Ankle Pull (Band Stretch)

This stretch will help loosen up the ankle.

Instructions:

- Sit on the floor with your legs straight out in front.
- Take a small towel or resistance and place it around your foot.
- Pull at the band, bringing your foot towards you.
- Hold for 10 seconds, then release, repeat the ten to fifteen times. Repeat on the other foot.

Toe Grip Challenges

This exercise will help to add strength to the muscles on your feet and toes.

Instructions:

- You can use something like a towel or a small object like marbles to help you with this.
- Place the object on the floor and try and grip it with your toes.
- Repeat this gripping motion at least ten times, then repeat on the other foot.

MASSAGE BALLS AND FOAM ROLLERS

I'm sure we have all experienced some sort of tightness in our muscles that makes us stiff and uncomfortable. This is not pleasant, and we want to get rid of this as quickly as possible so we can get our full range of motion back. Luckily there are a few tools that we can use to aid us in this. The massage ball and foam roller have been specifically designed to work out stiffness and knots in our muscles.

The connective tissue in your body that attaches your muscles, bones, and ligament is called fascia, and when they get tight, it is what usually causes this stiffness, you may be feeling. When this happens, knots and trigger points form that cause pain; the best way to get rid of them is to massage them out; this is called self-myofascial release. This is where the massage ball and foam rollers come in. If you don't want to go out and buy a massage ball, a tennis ball will work just fine.

Identify the area that has the knot or sore spot. Then, get either your ball or foam roller. You will want to lay down on the object or place it on a wall and gently rock back and forth over the knot; the pressure will help massage it out. Foam rollers work best for larger areas, and balls target very specific areas. Doing this regularly will prevent injuries and future discomfort. It is also an effective way to lengthen and warm up the muscles before stretching.

If you do have the budget to spend a bit more cash on something that will really benefit you through massages and getting out knots, then I would recommend getting a TheraGun. It uses a combination of force and vibrations to relieve pain and stiffness; it can also vastly increase your range of motion. It does all of this without you having to put in anywhere near as much effort as mentioned with massage balls, foam rollers.

3

REPETITIONS: STRETCHING ROUTINES THAT MAKE YOU RECOVER FASTER

M ost of us will have at least a few minor muscle injuries or sprains in our lifetime. These can come from exercise, general life, lack of flexibility, or an illness. It is pretty much inevitable, but there are specific routines that can help us overcome these faster, so we don't have to be stuck in that position for a long time.

ROUTINES FOR SPRAINS, INJURIES, ACHES AND PAINS

Minor injuries and sprains, while may not be very serious, can cause some problems and slow us down quite a bit. Let's take a look at a few routines that can help us recover from these specific injuries quicker.

Calf Routine

This is a common injury that occurs when you put too much force on your calf muscle or overstretch it. Take a look at the routine below that will help. You do not have to do all these at once, that might put too much strain on your muscle. Rather start with the first few and then keep adding on more exercises as you get stronger.

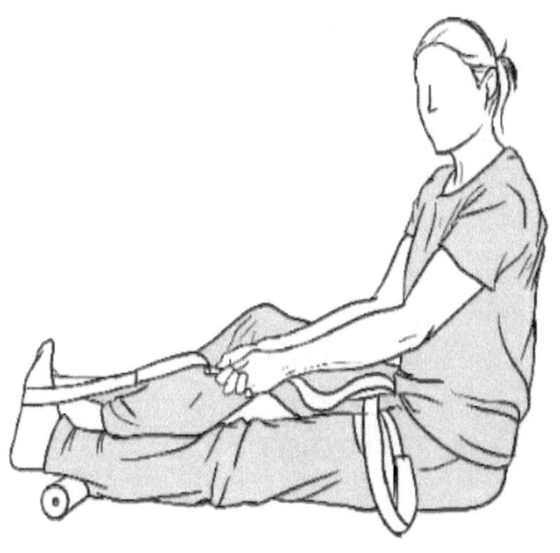

Calf Stretch 1:

- Sit down on the ground with your legs out in front of you.
- Place a roll or rolled-up towel under your ankle to elevate it.
- Grab a strap or belt and place it on your top part of your foot, just below the toes.
- Pull with the strap until you feel the stretch. You might feel a little bit of pain but not too much.
- Hold for 30 seconds and repeat three times.

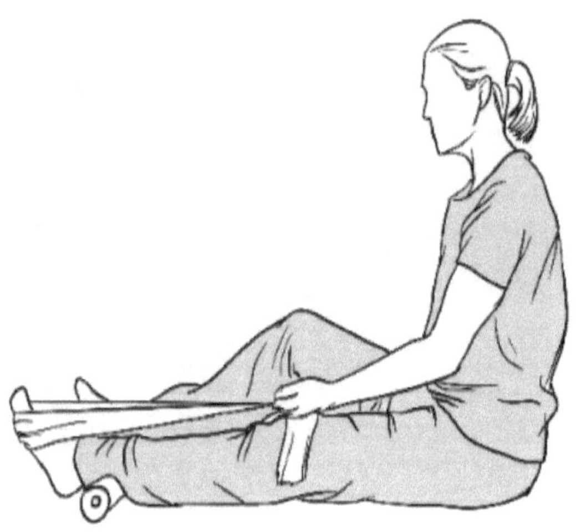

Calf Stretch 2:

- Grab a resistance band, choose the lowest resistance, and place that on the ball of your foot. The roll or towel is still under your ankle.
- Push your toes forward against the resistance band.
- Then slowly bring your foot back up, use controlled movements.
- Repeat ten times at first. If you can, then increase your reps to about fifteen or twenty.

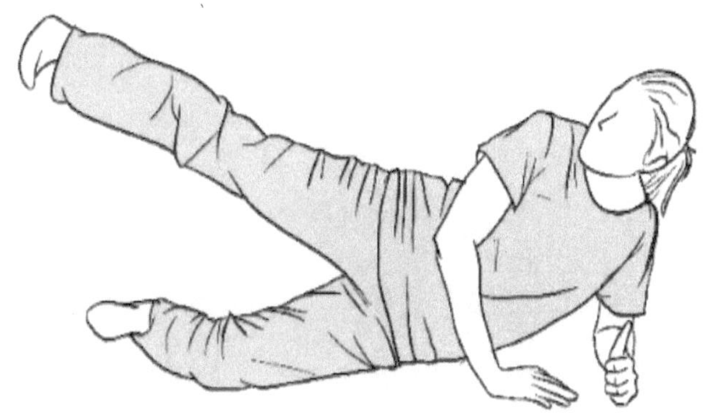

Calf Stretch 3:

- Lay down on your side, bend your bottom leg backward and lift your top leg slightly off the ground.
- Flex your foot, you should feel it in your calf. Point your toe slightly to the floor.
- Pick your leg up and back in one motion; you don't have to lift it too high.
- Bring your leg back down in one controlled movement.
- Start by doing ten to fifteen and then increase if it is easy for you. You may add some weights if you need something extra.

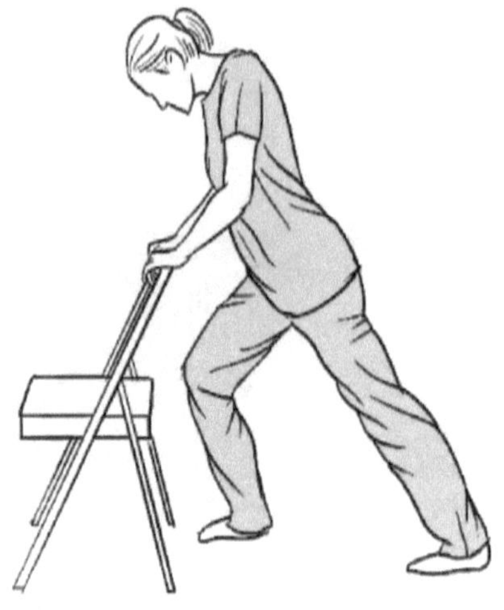

Calf Stretch 4:

- Grab a chair and hold onto the back.
- Take a step back with one leg so that it's stretched out behind you. The other leg should be slightly bent in front of you. Toes pointed forward.
- Lean into your front leg. Hold for 30 seconds and repeat three times.

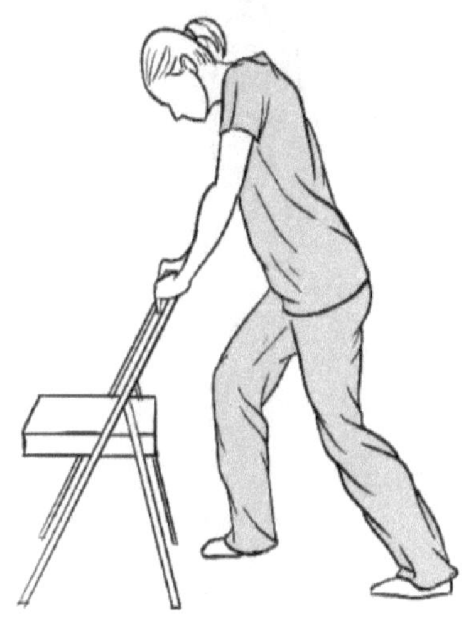

Calf Stretch 5:

- Start in the same position as the previous exercise, but instead of having a straight back leg, just bend it slightly.
- Then lean in and stretch out the muscle. This stretch targets the soleus muscle just below the calf, that's where you should feel it.
- Hold for 30 seconds and repeat three times.

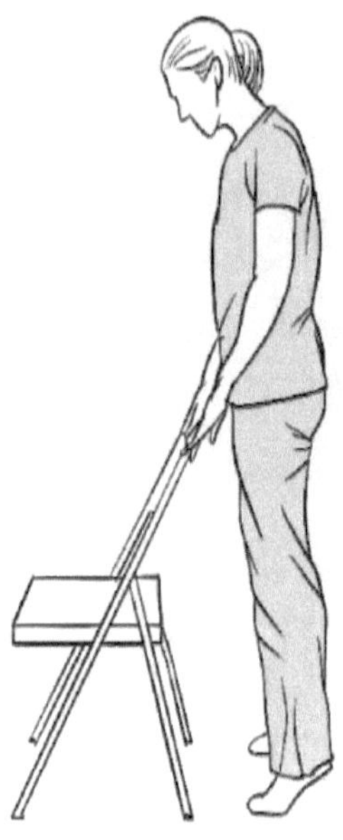

Calf Stretch 6:

- Follow the instructions for the Tip Toe Tense stretch mentioned in the previous chapter.
- Start with about ten repetitions and increase it if you feel you can.

The following exercises are a bit more intense, only do these towards the end of your recovery when you feel that your muscle has strengthened up a bit.

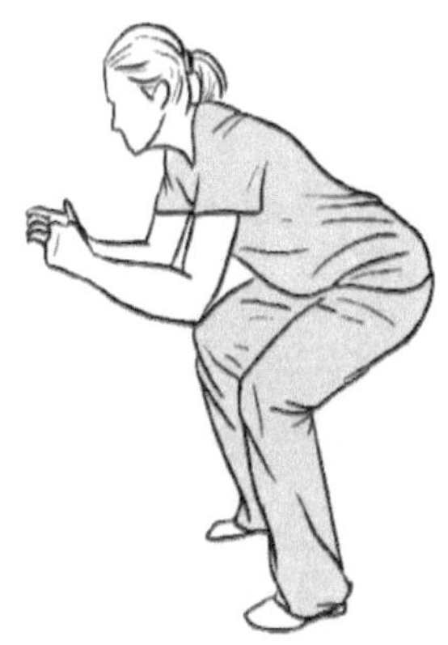

Calf Stretch 7:

- Get into a squat position and lower yourself down into a squat.
- When you bring yourself back up, extend the movement until you are on your toes.
- This should all be one controlled and fluid motion.
- Start with doing five and work your way up.

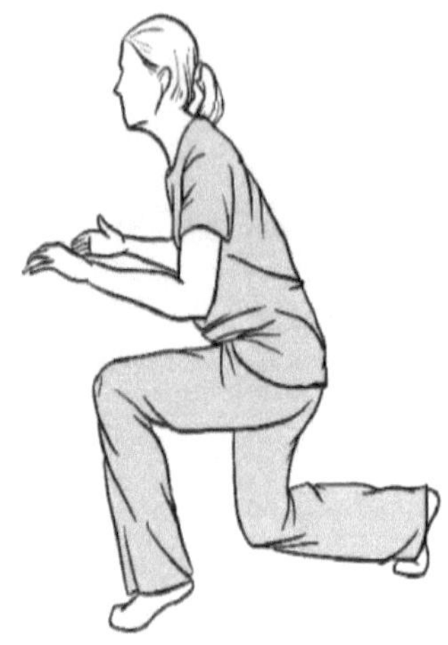

Calf Stretch 8:

- Get into a lunge position—one foot in front and the other behind.
- Get up on your toes on both feet.
- Bend your back knee down, and then bring yourself back up again.
- This should be in one fluid motion.
- Start with five, and when you are comfortable, increase the number you do.

Hamstring Routine

Hamstrings are a common muscle that can get quite tight and get pulled or injured during exercise. If you have a hamstring injury, then the following routine will help you to start recovering.

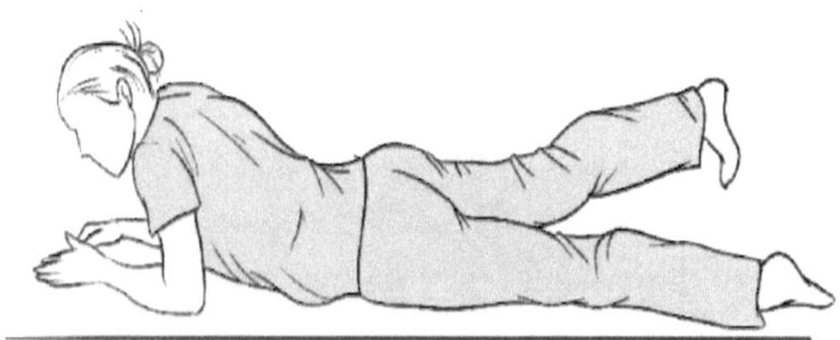

Hamstring Stretch 1:

- Lay down on your belly, prop your body up with your elbows.
- Lift one of your feet as high as you can and then lower it down in one smooth motion.
- Do about ten and see if you can increase it from there.

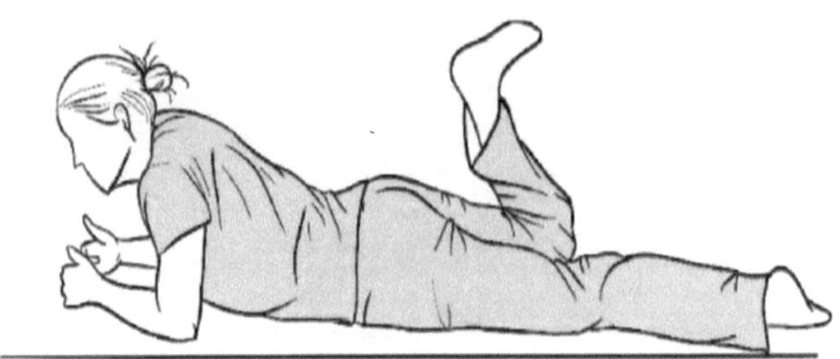

Hamstring Stretch 2:

- Stay on your belly and lift the foot so that it moves towards your butt.
- Keep the motion slow and controlled.
- Start with ten and then add on if you think you can do more.

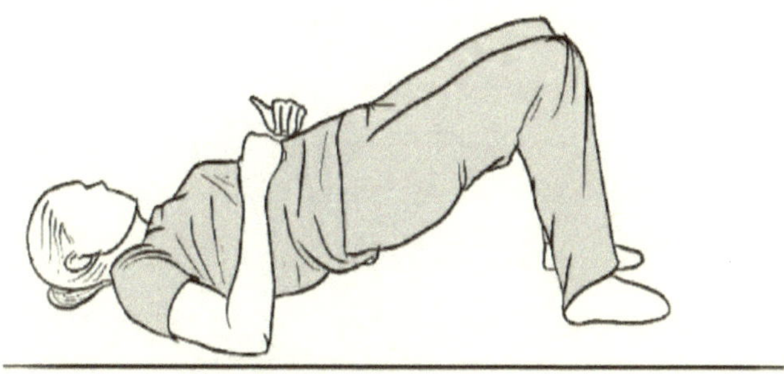

Hamstring Stretch 3:

- Roll over onto your back and bend your knees.
- Lift your hips off the ground and then slowly bring it down.
- Start with ten and then work your way up.
- Make it harder by completing the single-leg version

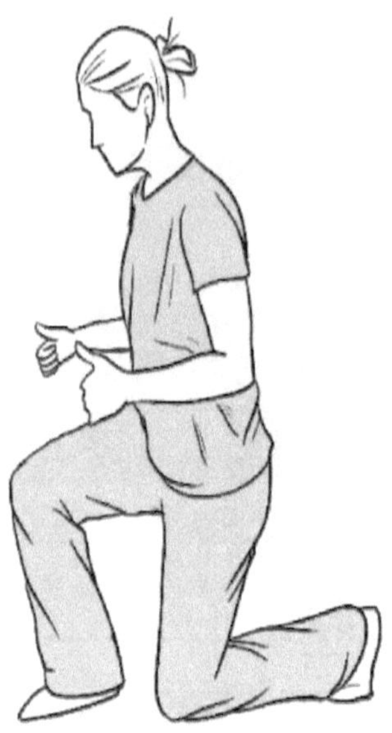

Hamstring Stretch 4:

- Get into a lunge position and just proceed to do a simple lunge.
- Bring your body down and up in one smooth movement, do this slowly.
- Do ten and then work your way up if you can.

Quad Routine

Quads usually get strained when too much force is exerted on it, often due to sports or inflexibility. If you have a pulled quad, do the following routine a few times a day until it heals up.

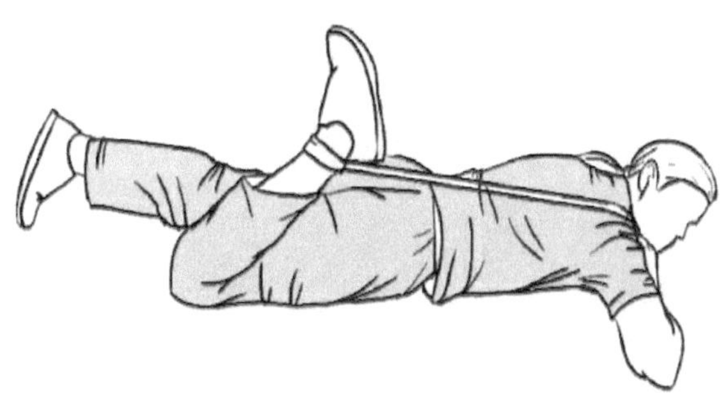

Quad Stretch 1:

- Lay down on your belly and either grab your ankle or use a belt to hold onto your ankle as you pull it towards your butt.
- Pull as far as you can, hold for 30 seconds. Repeat this three times.

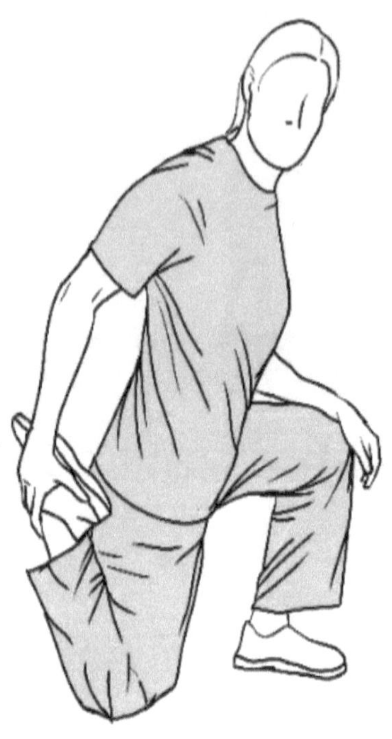

Quad Stretch 2:

- Get on your knees and place one foot in front of you, bent at a 90-degree angle.
- Grab your back foot and bring it up towards your butt, if you would like more of a stretch lean into your front leg.
- Hold for 30 seconds and repeat this three times.

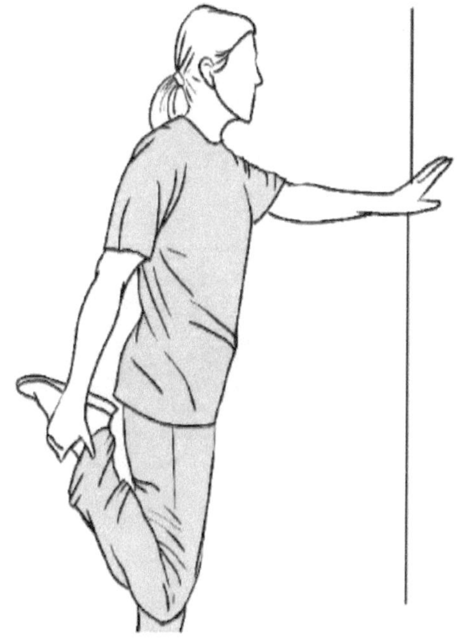

Quad Stretch 3:

- Stand up with your back straight.
- Bend the foot so that it moves toward your butt, grab the foot with your hand and pull it into your butt.
- Make sure both of your knees are still in line.
- Hold for 30 seconds and repeat three times.

Glute Strain

Glute strain can happen from too much sitting or exercising funny. If you have a strain on your glute muscles, follow this routine.

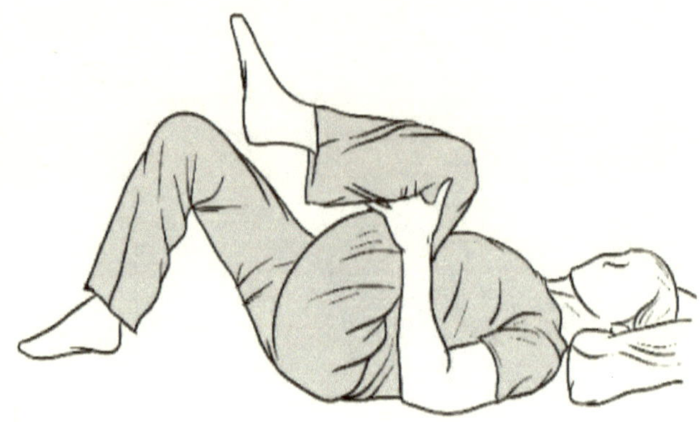

Glute Stretch 1:

- Lay down on your back with your knees bent, grab under your thigh and pull it closer to your body.
- You should feel the stretch in your glute.
- Hold for 30 seconds, repeat three times on each side.

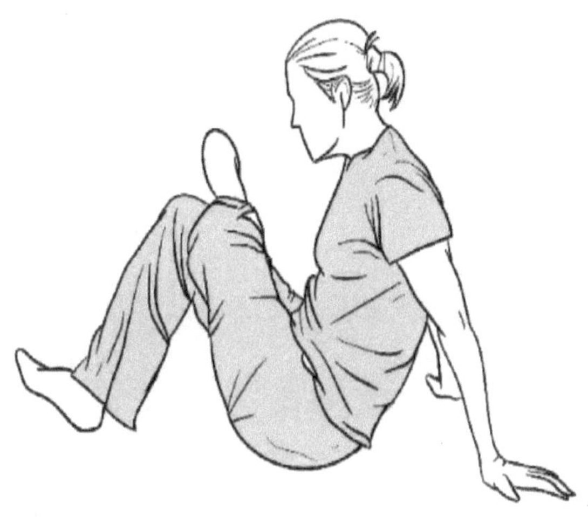

Glute Stretch 2:

- Follow the instructions for the Lying Figure 4 Stretch mentioned in the previous chapter.
- If you want more of a stretch instead of lying down, do it sitting up.
- Use your hands as support behind you and use the leg on the ground to move the bent leg closer to your chest.
- Hold for 30 seconds, repeat three times on each side.

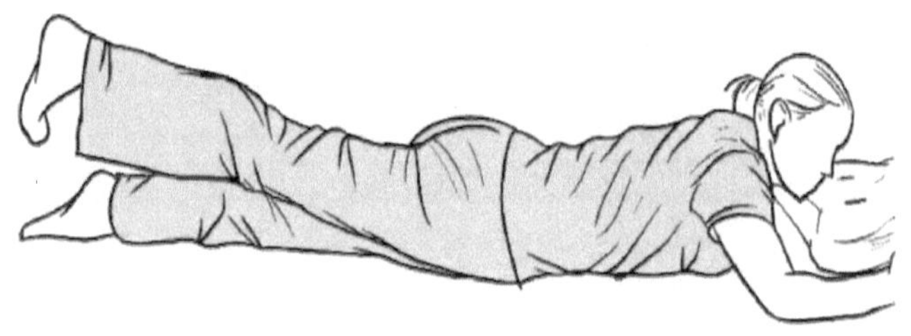

Glute Stretch 3:

- Lay down on your belly, squeeze your butt in tight.
- Lift your leg back.
- Hold for 3 seconds, relax and then repeat ten times.

Groin Strains

A groin strain is a strain on the adductor muscles in your legs. They are positioned in the inner thigh if you have a groin strain use the following routine.

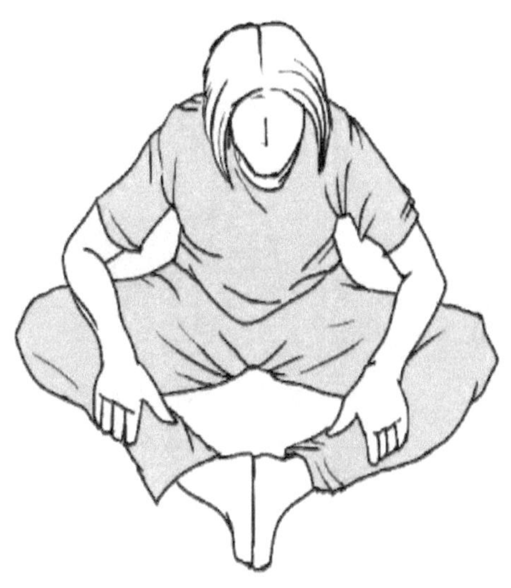

Groin Stretch 1:

- Sit down on the floor and bring your feet together, so the soles of the feet are touching.
- Take your elbows and push down on your inner thighs.
- Lean forward towards your feet.
- Hold for 30 seconds and repeat three times.
- If you want more of a stretch in your inner thigh, pull your feet closer to you.

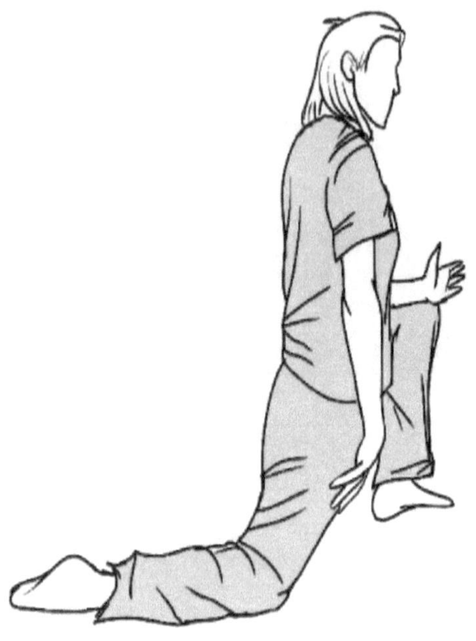

Groin Stretch 2:

- Get down on one knee with the other leg in front of you.
- Move that leg to the side, as far as it is comfortable for you.
- Push forward with your hips.
- Hold for 30 seconds and repeat three times on each leg.

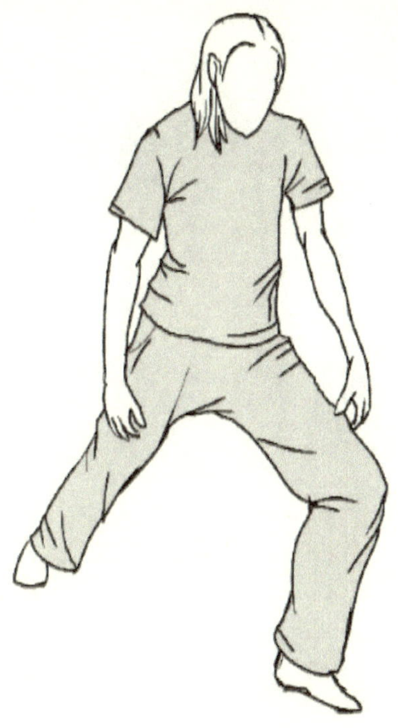

Groin Stretch 3:

- Stand up straight and step your foot forward and to the outside in a 45-degree angle.
- Push yourself forward into your front leg.
- Hold for 30 seconds and repeat three times.

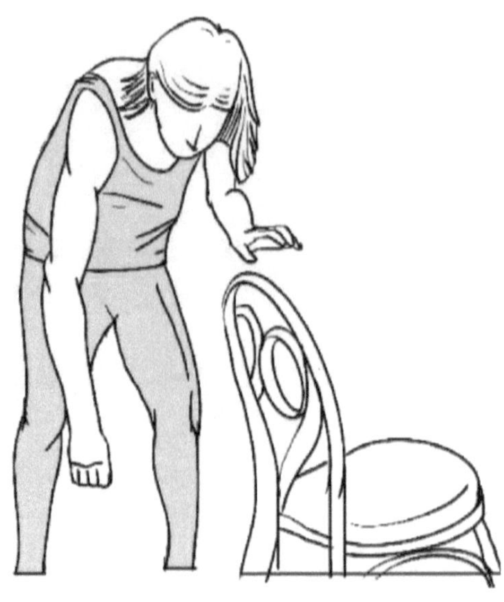

Shoulder Pain

If we put too much weight on our shoulders or funnily sleep on our shoulders, it can cause shoulder pain. If you suffer from shoulder pain, follow this routine.

Shoulder Stretch 1:

- Bend down and hold onto a chair, let your arm hang down in front of you.
- Swing your body around like a pendulum; your whole body should be moving, not just your arm.
- If you want your shoulder to open up a bit more, hold a weight in your hand.
- Do this for a few minutes.

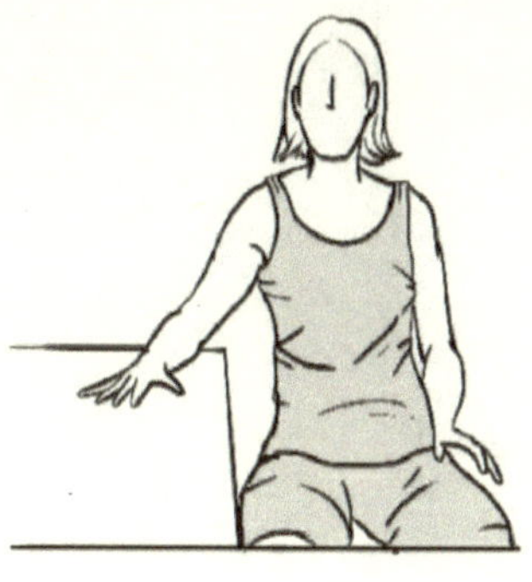

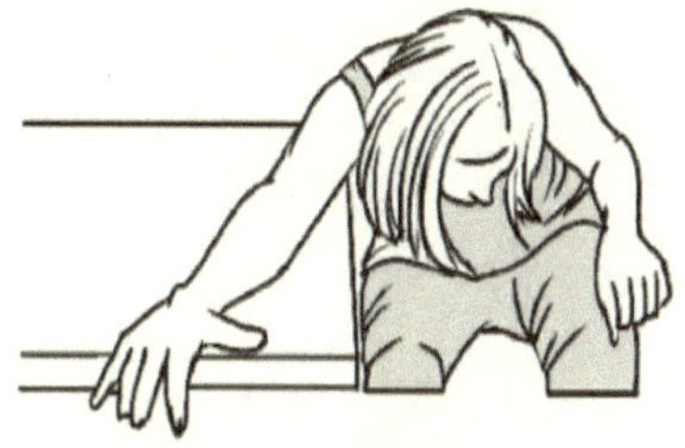

Shoulder Stretch 2:

- Sit at a table and place your forearm on the surface.
- Slide the arm forward and backward on the table to open up the shoulder.
- Then do the same movement at a 45-degree angle on the table.
- Move on to sliding in circles if those feel good.
- Repeat as many times as desired.

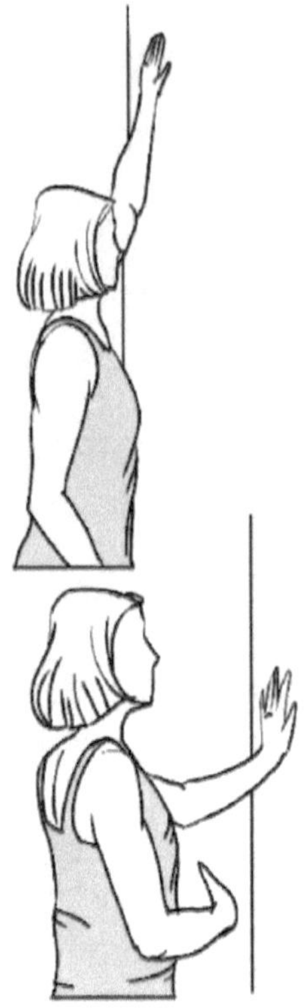

Shoulder Stretch 3:

- Place your hand on a wall.
- Slide it up and once you get pretty high lean into the wall.
- Bring your hand back down.
- Repeat as many times as desired.

Rotator Cuff Stain

The rotator cuff surrounds the shoulder and is made up of muscles and tendons. If you have injured your rotator cuff, then follow this routine. You may also incorporate the shoulder routine above and vice versa.

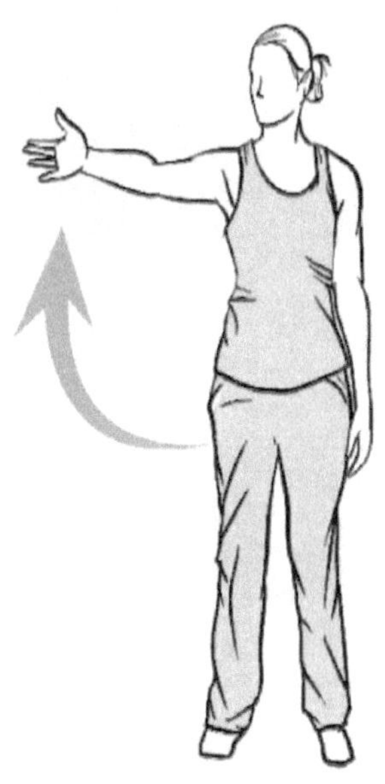

Rotator Cuff Stretch 1:

- Stand up straight with your arm just slightly in front of you facing 45 degrees to the side.
- With a straight arm, lift it to about 90 degrees and bring it down again.
- Use controlled movements.
- Repeat as many times as desired.

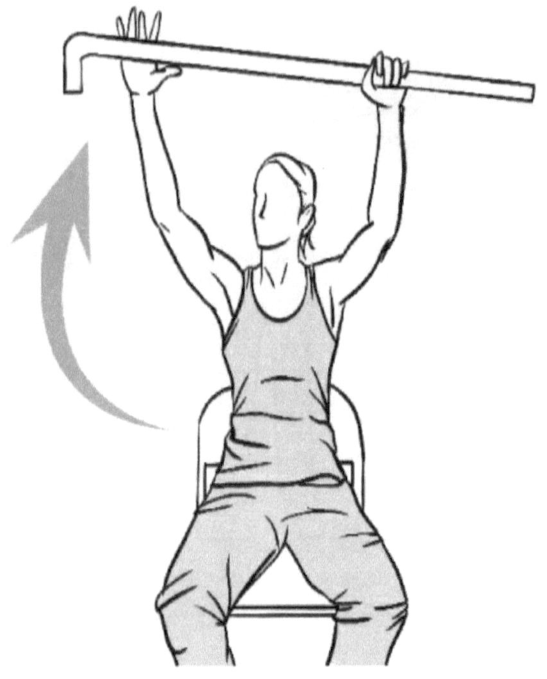

Rotator Cuff Stretch 2:

- Sit down on a chair and have either a stick or a pipe in hand.
- The injured side is just going to rest on the stick, and the other hand will be doing all the work.
- Place the hand of the injured side on the stick, lift the stick with the other hand until it is just over your head.
- Slowly bring it back down.
- Repeat as many times as desired.

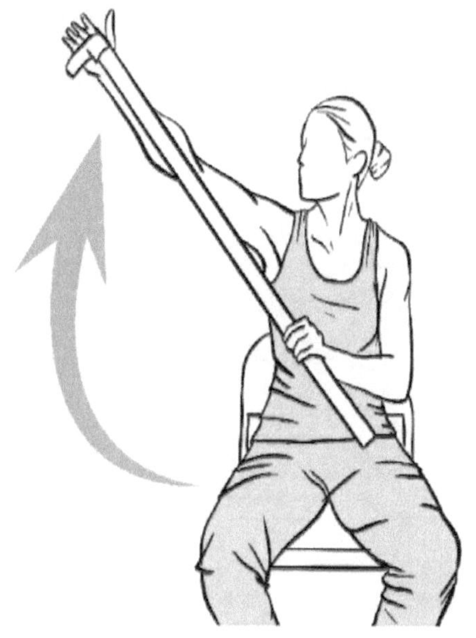

Rotator Cuff Stretch 3:

- This is the same principle as stretch 2. The injured hand is just resting while the other one is doing the work.
- Place the hand of the injured arm on the side of the stick or pipe and use your other hand to push it to the side.
- Repeat as many times as desired.

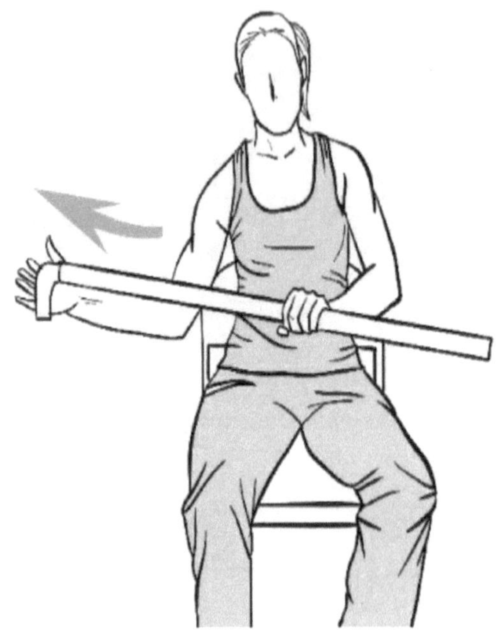

Rotator Cuff Stretch 4:

- Still using the pipe or stick, hold the hand of your injured side at a 90-degree angle with your fingers facing forward.
- Use the pipe or stick to push the hand back. The motion is the same as that of a door opening and closing.
- Repeat as many times as desired.

You may also want to refer to the shoulder pain exercises.

Knee and Hip Strain

Knee and hip injuries can occur for many different reasons, but they can be quite debilitating if not attended to. Use the following routine to ease any discomfort in these areas.

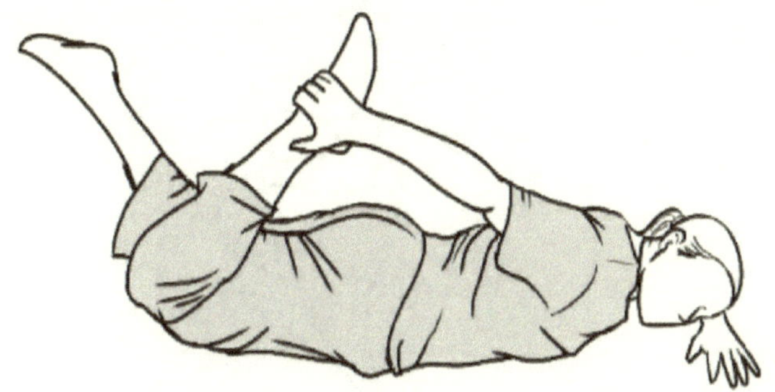

Knee and Hip Stretch 1:

- Lay down on the ground with your belly facing the floor.
- Put your face down on the ground and take your arm around your back to grab your foot.
- Pull your leg up off the ground; your shoulder can be off the ground as well.
- Hold for 30 seconds and repeat three times.

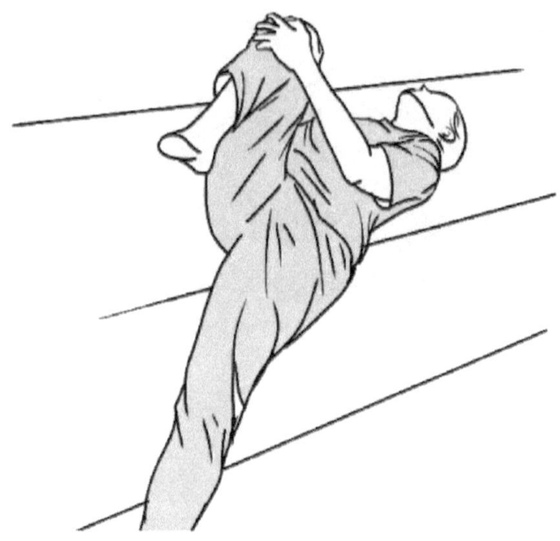

Knee and Hip Stretch 2:

- Lay down on the edge of a bed. Your injured side should be hanging off the side of the bed. Be careful that you don't slip off.
- Grab the shin of your other leg and pull it into your body.
- This stretch allows the hip to stretch using its natural weight.
- Hold for 30 seconds and repeat three times.

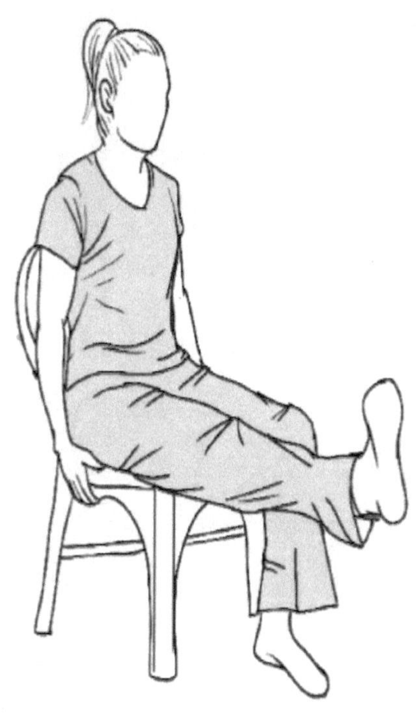

Knee and Hip Stretch 3:

- Sit on a chair with your back straight. You shouldn't be leaning back during this stretch.
- Slowly kick your leg straight out and slowly bring it back down to the ground.
- If it is too easy for you, add some weight to your ankle
- Repeat ten to fifteen times and increase as you get stronger.

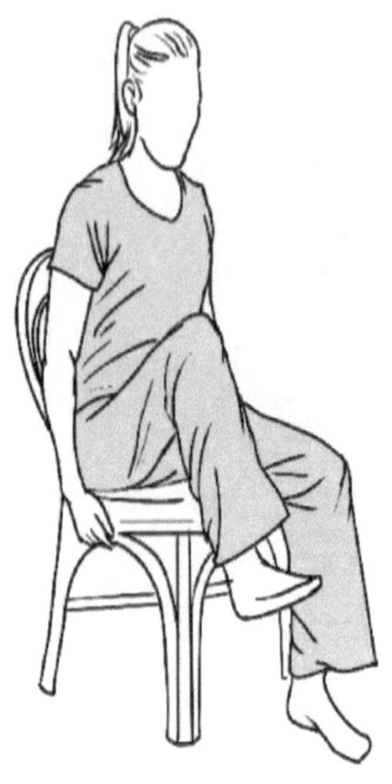

Knee and Hip Stretch 4:

- Still sitting on your chair, drive your knee up.
- Slowly bring it down. Make sure your movements are controlled.
- This is a hip flexion strengthening move.
- Do this ten to fifteen times and increase as you get stronger.

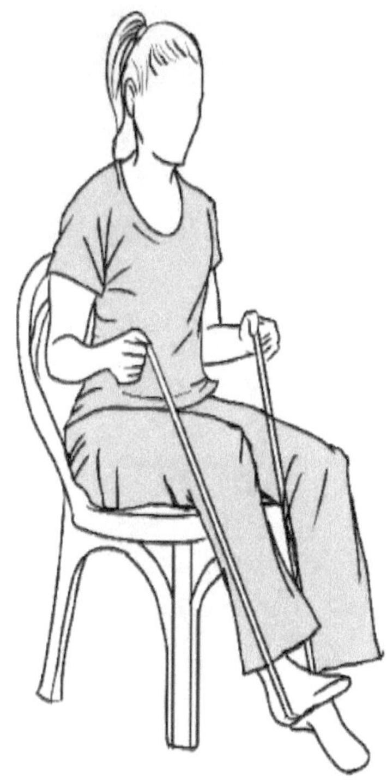

Knee and Hip Stretch 5:

- Grab a resistance band, use the band that is the lowest resistance.
- Place the band in the middle of your foot.
- With controlled movements, lift your knee up and then push down into the resistance band.
- Repeat ten to fifteen times and increase as you get stronger.

Achilles Pain

The Achilles tendon is the tissue that connects the calf muscle to the heel bone. When we have pain in this area, especially if it's constant, it is called Achilles tendinitis. Follow this routine to help stretch out this area and get it feeling better.

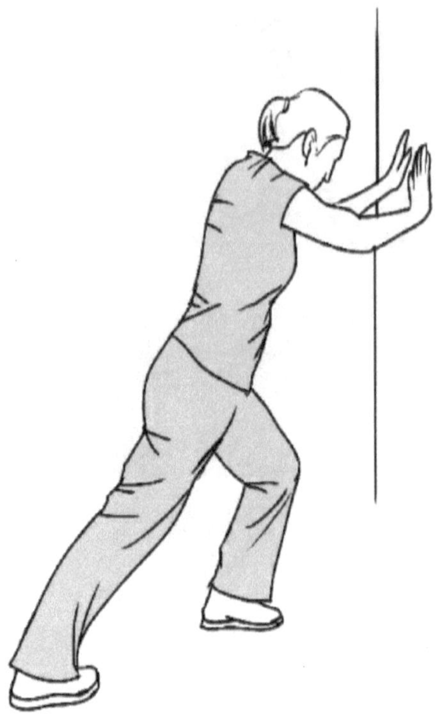

Achilles Stretch 1:

- Start by standing next to a wall; you will be leaning against it.
- Step forward with one leg and have the other one behind you. The leg behind you will be the one being stretched out.
- Make sure your feet are faced towards the wall and are flat on the ground.
- Bend your front left and lean into that leg, so it moves towards the wall. Keep your back leg straight.
- Hold for 30 seconds and repeat three times.

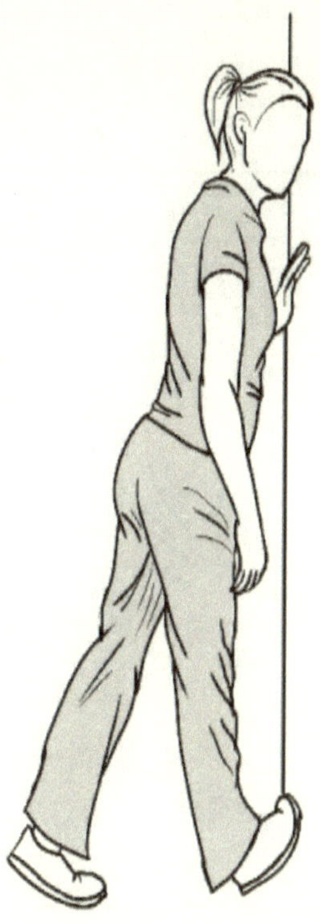

Achilles Stretch 2:

- Get up close to the wall and place your toes on the wall.
- Get your toes as high as you can on the wall while your heel is still on the ground.
- Lean into the wall with your body.
- Hold this for 30 seconds and repeat three times.

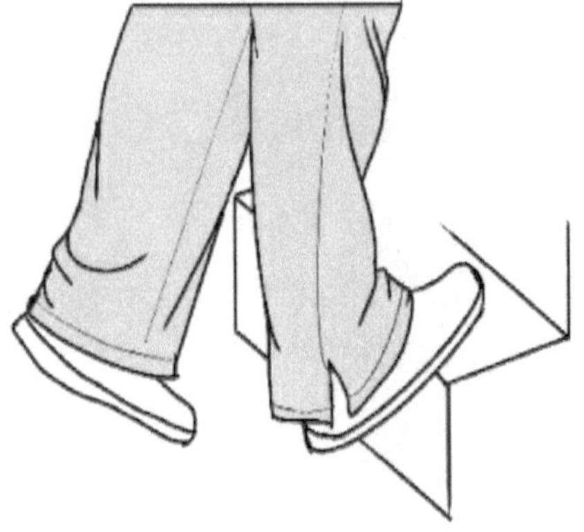

Achilles Stretch 3:

- You will need a step or step ladder for this stretch.
- Place the ball of your foot onto the step and let your heel hang off. Your other foot should also be hanging off the step.
- Drop the heel of your foot as low as you can get it; you will feel the stretch in your Achilles tendon.
- Hold this for 30 seconds and repeat three times.

Back Strains

Many things can cause back strains from lifting heavy weights to having improper posture or even just sleeping in an uncomfortable position. If you have a back strain, then follow this routine to ease that pain.

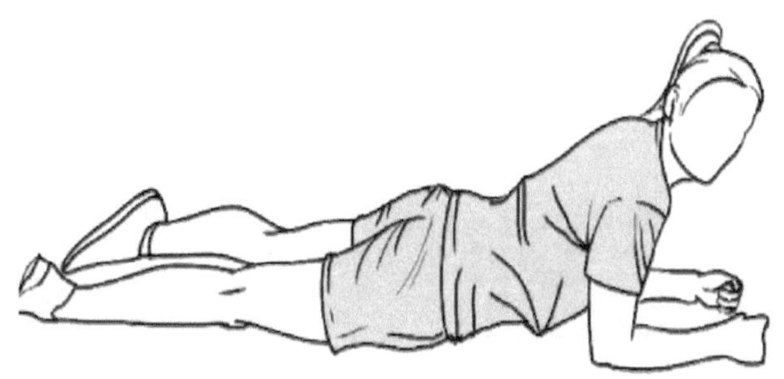

Back Stretch 1:

- Lay down on your belly and prop yourself up on your elbows.
- Your hips should be on the ground, try not to lift your stomach either.
- Hold this position for 30 seconds and repeat three times.

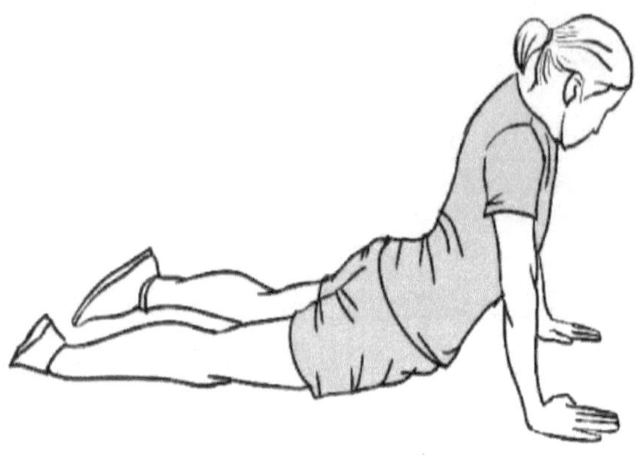

Back Stretch 2:

- This is just a step further from the previous one.
- Lift yourself on your hands, try and keep your hips to the ground.
- Hold this for 30 seconds and repeat three times.

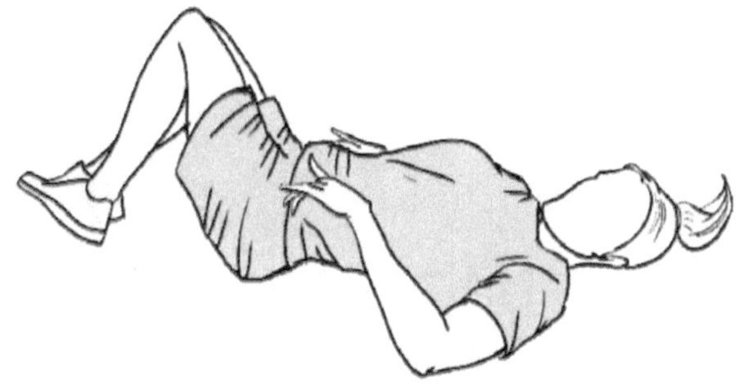

Back Stretch 3:

- Move over onto your back, have your knees pointing to the ceiling.
- Drop your knees to the one side and roll your hips over, before your knees touch the ground start rolling over to the other side.
- Do this ten times or hold for 30 seconds and repeat three times.

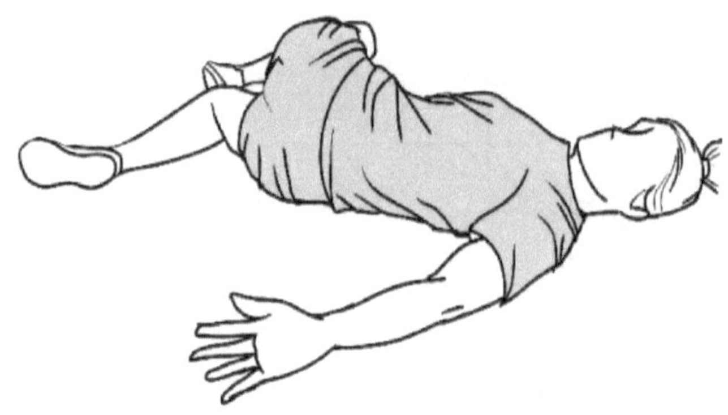

Back Stretch 4:

- This is the next progression from Back Stretch 3.
- When you roll over to one side, drop your knee to the ground and pull it up to a 90-degree angle and drop it to the ground.
- If you want a deeper stretch in your lumbar, take your hand and press down on your top leg.
- Hold for 30 seconds and repeat on the other side.

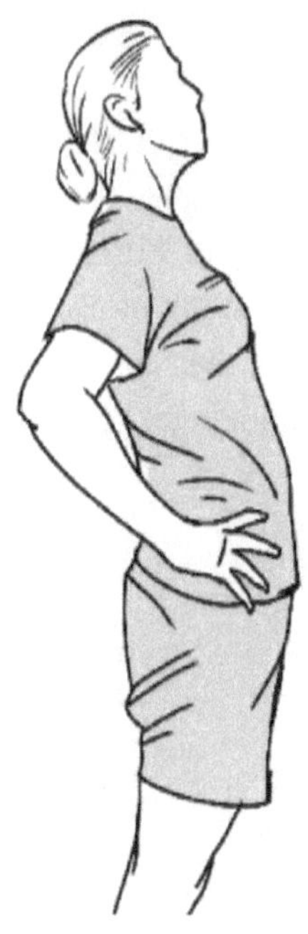

Back Stretch 5:

- Stand up straight and place your hands on your hips.
- Rotate your hips back so that you are looking at the ceiling, the hands-on your hips should give you some support. Don't bend your knees.
- Hold for 30 seconds and repeat three times.

MOBILITY LIMITING ILLNESSES

Joint and muscle pain are most commonly caused by the things we do in our daily lives, but in some cases, pain is caused by illnesses. These illnesses show up usually by no fault of our own; they are just age or genetics. While there may not be anything that we can do to stop ourselves from getting these illnesses, there is something we can do to reduce discomfort significantly. These stretching routines will help ease the discomfort and strengthen the joints and muscles so that you can live a more comfortable life.

Arthritis

Arthritis is pretty common, mostly in older people, but it has been seen in people who are teens and young adults as well. It is most common in the hands, and it can cause joint pain and stiffness. Sometimes it causes redness and swelling in the joint areas. You might also notice your range of mobility has lessened. If you have arthritis, then follow this routine to help relieve the pressure on your joints and strengthen up your hands in the process.

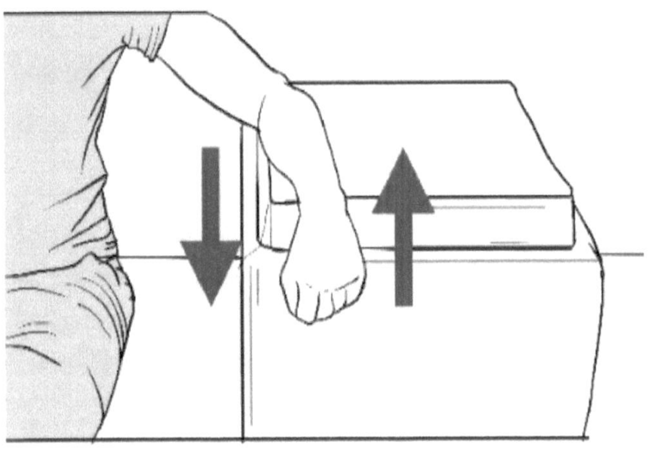

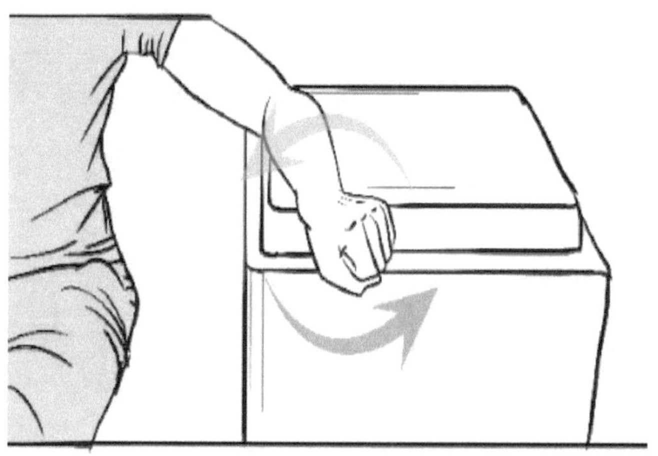

Arthritis Stretch 1:

- Prop your arm up on a table or counter. Let your wrist hang off the edge.
- Warm your wrist up by moving it up and down on the edge of the counter. Do this about ten to fifteen times.
- Switch to moving your wrist side to side, also ten to fifteen times.

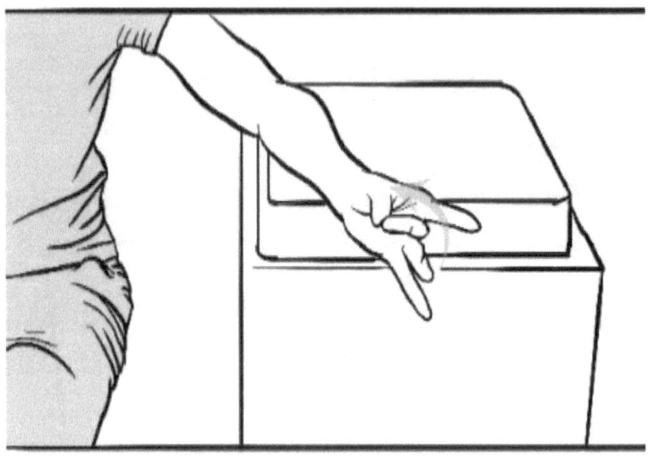

Arthritis Stretch 2:

- Open up your hands like you are showing the number 5.
- Keep your fingers as straight as possible and bring your fingers in one by one to meet your thumb. This allows the focus to be on the bottom joints of the fingers.
- Repeat this about three times on all your fingers.

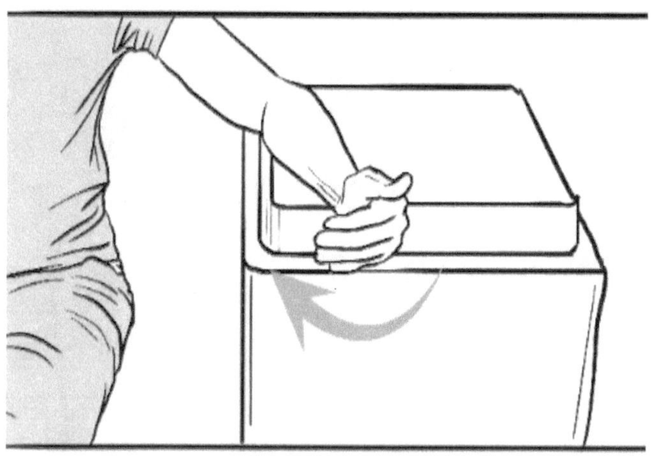

Arthritis Stretch 3:

- Still, with your hand open, stick all your fingers together with the thumb facing up.
- Keeping your fingers straight, bend at the knuckle to try and create a 90-degree angle with your hand. Release and go back to a straight hand.
- Next, focus on the joint just above your knuckle. Bend that in, almost creating a claw. Release and go back to the starting position.
- Next, move to the top joint of the finger. You also want just to move this joint down, this can be difficult, so hold your finger just below the joint and move it down. Do this with each finger.
- Repeat each one of these ten to fifteen times.

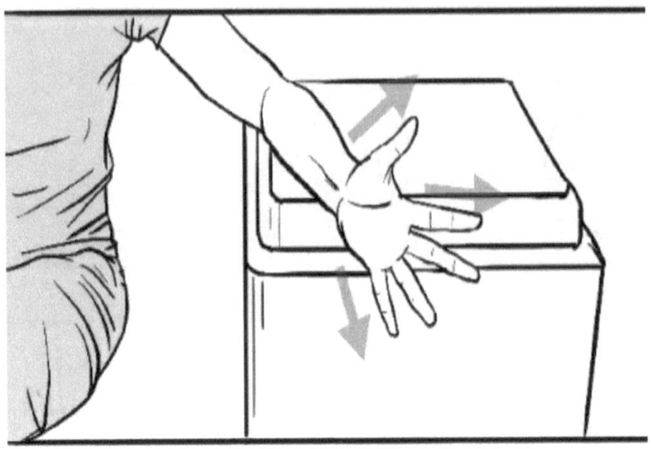

Arthritis Stretch 4:

- Start with your hand open and all your fingers together.
- Fan them out wide, then bring them back together.
- Do this for about 2 minutes a few times a day.
- You may repeat all the stretches in this routine a few times a day to ease any discomfort.

Tendonitis

The inflammation of the tendon causes tendonitis; it is more common in certain people than others. This is just due to genetics or the strain that is being placed on the tendon. If you put too much pressure or use the tendon too much, it can result in tendonitis. If you have tendonitis in your heel, you may follow the routine for stretching out the Achilles tendon that was mentioned above. If you have tendonitis in your wrist, then follow the following routine.

Tendonitis Stretch 1:

- The first stretch in this routine is the same one for Arthritis Stretch 1.
- Do these movements but do them slower and more controlled; you want to feel the stretch in the wrist.
- Do this ten to fifteen times.
- As you get stronger, you can do this with weight. Try a soup can or similar and do the same movements but while holding the can.

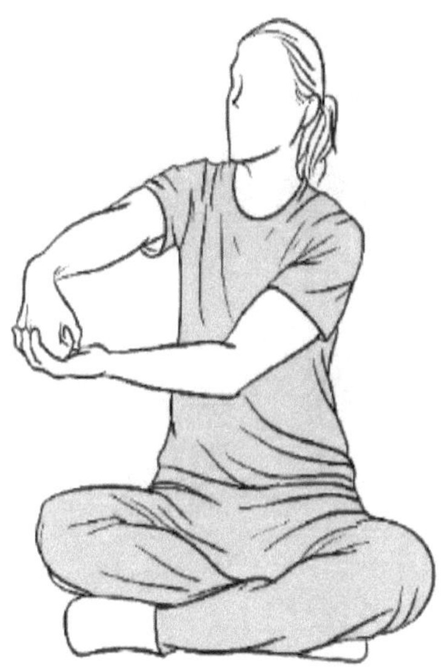

Tendonitis Stretch 2:

- Stretch out your arm in front of you and ball up your fist.
- Bend your wrist downwards and take your other hand and pull it towards you.
- Hold for 30 seconds.
- Open up your hands and flip your wrist upwards.
- Take the other hand, and pull the wrist towards you.
- Hold for 30 seconds.
- Repeat three times each way.
- Another variation would be to put your hands on the ground or wall and lean into it each way. You should feel all these stretches in your wrists and the tendons running up your forearms.

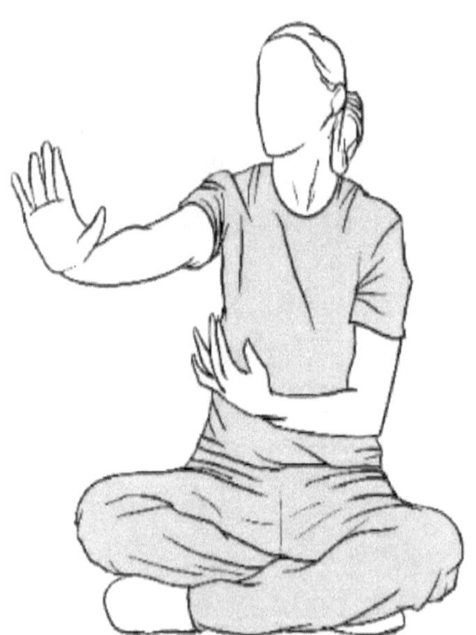

Tendonitis Stretch 3:

- Open up your hands so that your fingers are splayed out.
- Then ball it up into a fist. Repeat as many times as desired.
- You do not need to hold this; the goal is just to get your hand moving.

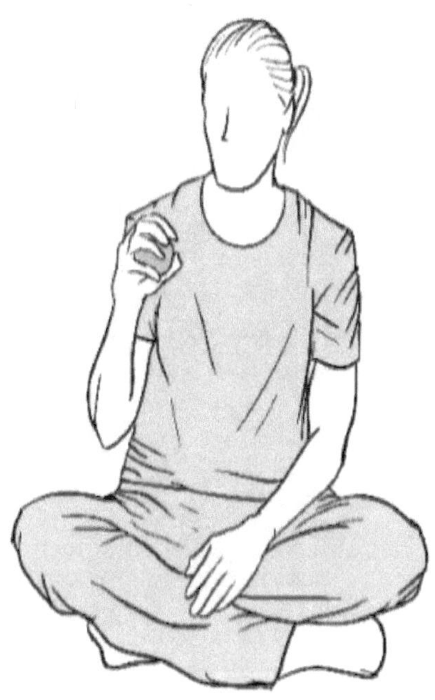

Tendonitis Stretch 4:

- Grab either a stress ball or a tennis ball.
- Squeeze that in your hands for about five to ten seconds.
- Release and repeat five times.
- If you don't have a ball or want something softer, you can use a pool noodle or rolled-up towel.

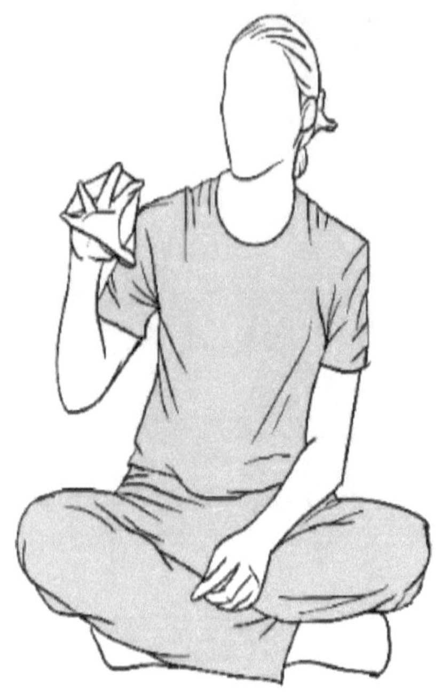

Tendonitis Stretch 5:

- Grab a small rubber band.
- Place it around your fingers and stretch your fingers open and closed.
- Go slow, so the band doesn't pop off.
- You want to repeat this about three times.

Carpal Tunnel Syndrome

Carpal tunnel syndrome is found in the arm and wrist and is a result of a pinched nerve. The symptoms are usually tingling, sensitivity, pain, and numbness. If you suffer from carpal tunnel syndrome, then follow this routine to ease discomfort and pain.

You should feel stretching and tension when doing these stretches, but not any severe pain. You might feel tingling in your fingertips; when you let it up, it should stop. If the tingling does not stop, this is an indication you have gone too far with the stretch. There is too much pressure on the nerve. Also, it might be an indication that there is something else wrong; this would be a good time to check in with your doctor or physician so they can diagnose you accurately.

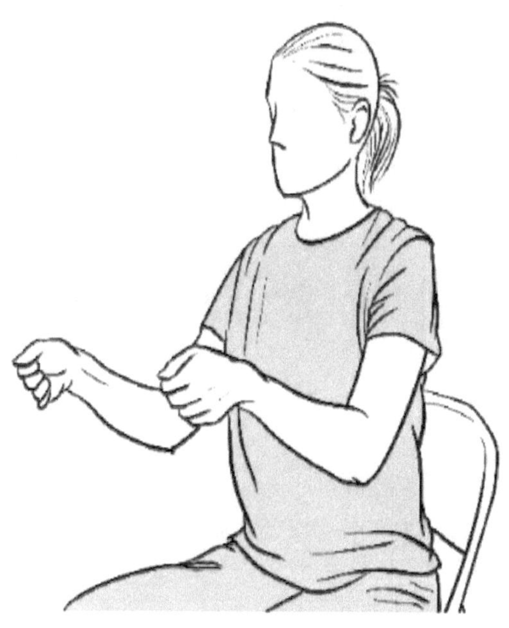

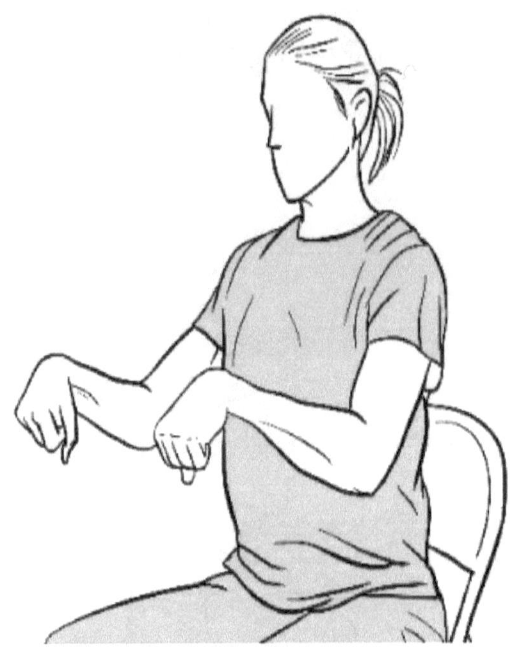

Carpal Tunnel Stretch 1:

- Hold your hands up in front of you, with your fists closed.
- Turn your wrists up, so your knuckles face the ceiling then bring them down to face the floor.
- Repeat ten times up and ten times down.
- Turn your hands to the side, so your thumb is upwards.
- Move your wrist up and then down, if the same motion as before.
- Repeat ten times up and ten times down.
- Make sure you are doing this is a continuous motion.

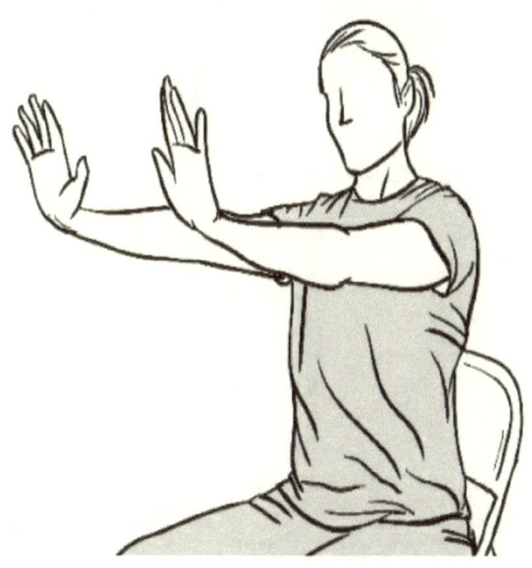

Carpal Tunnel Stretch 2:

- Stretch your arms out straight in front of you. Your hands should be open.
- Turn your wrists up so that your fingers point upwards.
- If you need less of a stretch, close your fingers. If you want more of a stretch, push your hands up against a wall.
- Hold for 30 seconds and repeat three times.

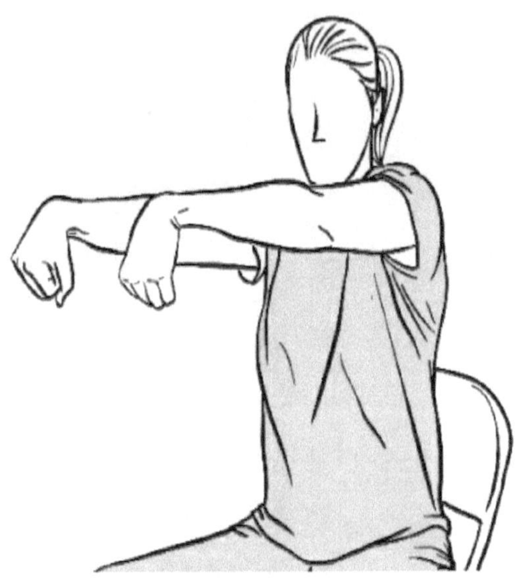

Carpal Tunnel Stretch 3:

- Still have your arms stretched out in front of you. Flip your wrists downward and curl your fingers in.
- If you want less of a stretch, then open up your fingers. If you want more of a stretch, then press your hands up against a wall.
- Hold for 30 seconds and repeat three times.

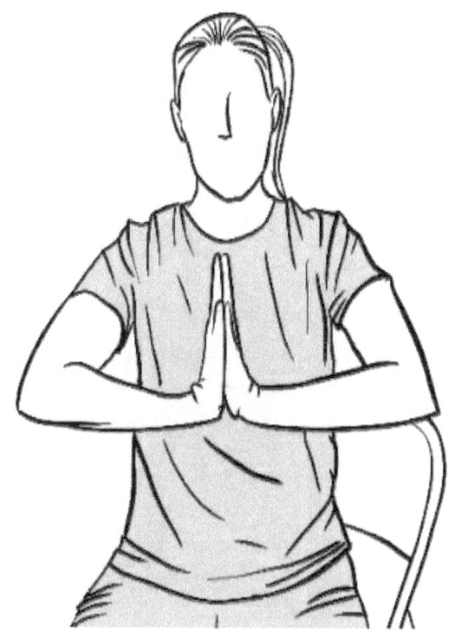

Carpal Tunnel Stretch 4:

- Place your palms together in a praying formation.
- Bring your wrists down, and at the same time, your elbows should be moving outwards.
- Push down as low as you can.
- Hold for 30 seconds and repeat three times.

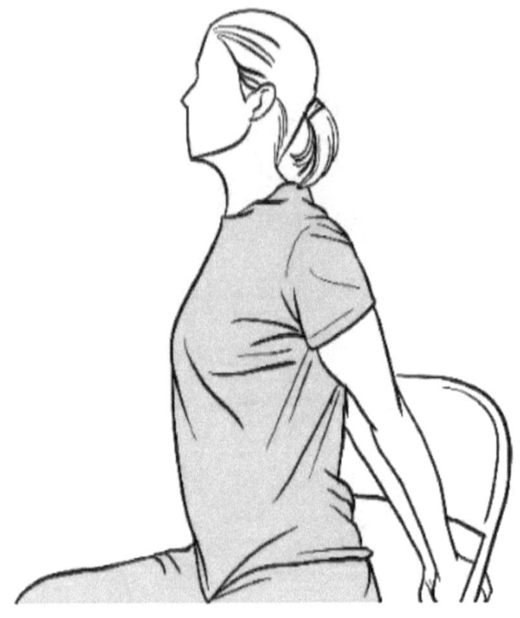

Carpal Tunnel Stretch 5:

- Clasp your hands behind you.
- Push your hands down and push your chest out.
- Hold for 30 seconds and repeat three times.
- This is more of a peck stretch, but it is good because that whole area is connected, so it would still be beneficial to you.

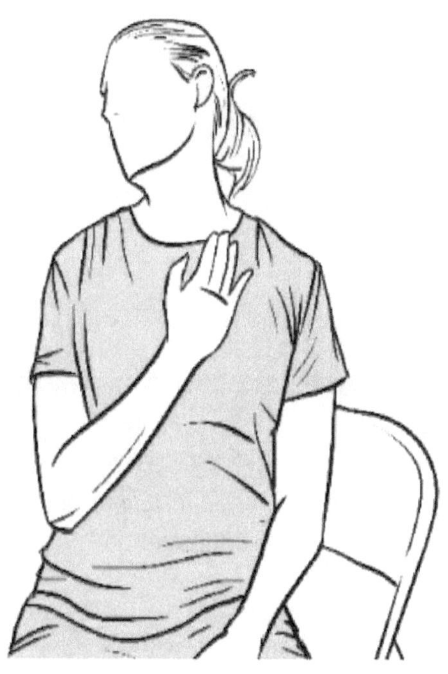

Carpal Tunnel Stretch 6:

- Hold your hand up to the side of your chest on a 90-degree angle.
  Your hand should be almost parallel to your head.
- Keep pressure on your upper chest and tilt your head the opposite side
  to your hand.
- Repeat ten times. Do this on the other side.
- This stretch is done to glide the nerve out, and it is not necessary to
  do it multiple times a day, since it could irritate the area.

4

THE FINAL PUSH: STRETCHING ROUTINES TO OPTIMIZE YOUR WORKOUTS

We have already chatted about the many benefits stretching has for your body and general life. But it can really improve the quality of your workouts as well. When you work out, your muscles are constantly flexing and contracting; they are in a constant state of movement. If you have limited flexibility, you will have limited muscle movement, which will put a cap on your workouts and progress.

Stretching also increases your rate of recovery after a workout. When we stretch, we increase blood circulation; this results in more nutrients being available for the muscles and a faster removal of harmful waste. You will ultimately feel better because of this. Stretching also provides you with a wider range of motion, which means the moves you perform can be more dynamic. No matter how far along you are in your fitness journey, stretching is a good weapon to have in your arsenal to increase your athletic development.

Using stretching in tandem with a workout is an extremely effective way to stay young and healthy. They tend to feed into each other; stretching improves your workouts or exercise, and that improves your health, and the cycle can then repeat.

GET THE MOST OUT OF YOUR STRETCH

As an athlete or avid gym-goer, you want to be able to get the most out of everything you do, and as with everything there is a right way and a wrong way to stretch. To reap all the benefits from stretching, you need to be mindful of a few things. The first thing is that stretching causes tension but not pain. That hurts so good feeling is normal; this shows that you are engaging those muscles, but any uncomfortable or piercing pain is an indication that you should stop. Pain can either be an indication that you have done the stretch wrong or that your muscles are not ready for that move as yet. Flexibility is built up over time, so don't rush it.

The second thing to remember is to breathe. Sometimes when we are so focused on the exercise or stretch, we forget that we need to breathe, when we hold our breath, our muscles tense up. We want our muscles to be as loose as possible when stretching, so remember to inhale and exhale constantly.

The third thing you need to keep in mind when it comes to stretching is that it is not a warm-up. In fact, your muscles should be warmed up for you to get the best out of your stretches. Cold muscles limit your movement and might even lead to injuries. The best way to warm up your muscles is a light 5 to 10-minute jog, either outside or on a treadmill. This will start activating your muscles and get them ready for your routine.

The final thing to remember when stretching is that you should not be bouncing. Stretching is about fluid motions, not stop-start or pulsing movements. Stretching is usually measured by the seconds you hold it for rather than how many you do, so if you are moving too quickly so that you can get to the next one, you will not get the most out of your stretch. Try and move as smoothly as possible; remember to relax and enjoy the moments.

ROUTINES FOR TARGETED AREAS

Every part of your body is different, and when it comes to stretching, each one has different requirements and a varied range of motion. I have broken up the stretching routines into sections; you will be able to partner stretching routines with the parts of your body you are working out that day. This way, you will be able to get the best results from your stretching and your workouts.

After each routine, you are encouraged to take a few minutes to connect with your body, engaging in a time of mindfulness. You can do this by lying down on your back and taking deep breaths. Think about how you feel and how the stretches made the different parts of your body feel. You may even find it helpful to touch the areas you are thinking about physically. The goal here is to increase the mind-body connection. If you know your body, you will be able to pick up on things faster.

Upper Body Routine

Having tight shoulders or a tight chest will diminish your range of motion, and you will lose some of the quality of your workout. Flexibility will help you get better results in any section of your upper body. They are all connected, and that is why it is essential not to neglect stretching out your entire upper body. Follow this routine to help you benefit from the flexibility of your upper body.

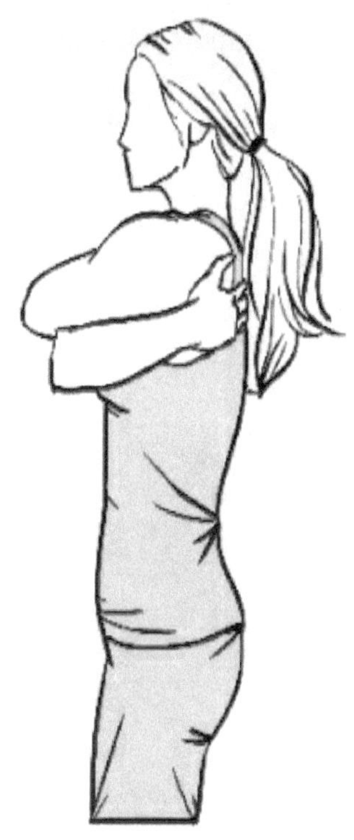

1. Self-hug Stretch

- Relax your shoulders. Take each of your hands and grab the opposite shoulder.
- Your arms should be one on top of the other and create a V shape on your chest. Your hands should be placed more to the side of the shoulder, not on top.
- Drop your shoulders down as far as you can get them while still keeping your eyes in front of you. Tuck your chin in.
- Let your chin drop towards your chest so that you will be moving your eyes towards the ground. Your chin should still be tucked.
- You should feel the stretch in the middle-upper part of your back. As soon as you feel the stretch, hold it for five breaths. Your shoulders should not be moving when you breathe.

This stretch lengthens the upper part of your back. If your back is very straight, this could compromise how your neck mechanics work; this stretch will loosen this up by introducing a slight forward arch. Loosened back and neck will reduce the risk of injury when you are lifting heavyweights.

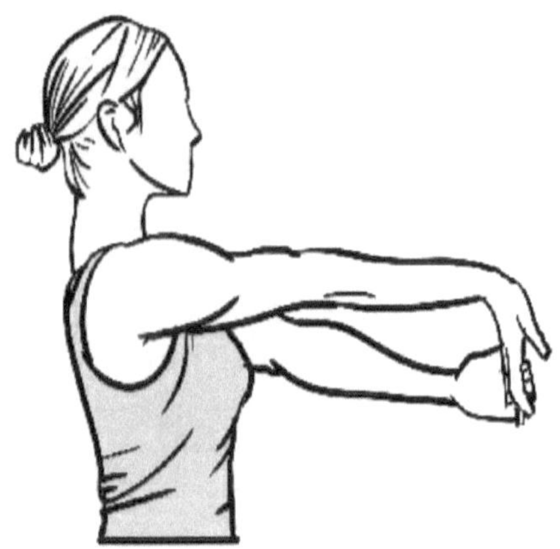

2. Forearm Stretch

- Stretch your arms out straight in front of you.
- Flip your wrist up so that your fingers are pointing to the ceiling.
- Take one of your hands and pull back the fingers of the other hand.
- You should feel this stretch both in your wrist and the inner part of your forearm.
- Hold for 30 seconds.
- Next, flip your wrist downwards and curl your fingers in.

- With the other hand, pull the curled hand towards you.
- You will feel the stretch running up the back of the forearm.
- Hold for 30 seconds.
- Repeat this stretch three times each on both sides.

Stretching your forearms can often be overlooked, but this stretch stretches both the forearm and the fingers. You need your forearms to lift and your finger flexon to grip. After a long day of not using the forearm muscles, they become tight and shrink. Most jobs do not require the use of the forearm muscle, so it is our responsibility to make sure this muscle is engaged, so it has good mobility.

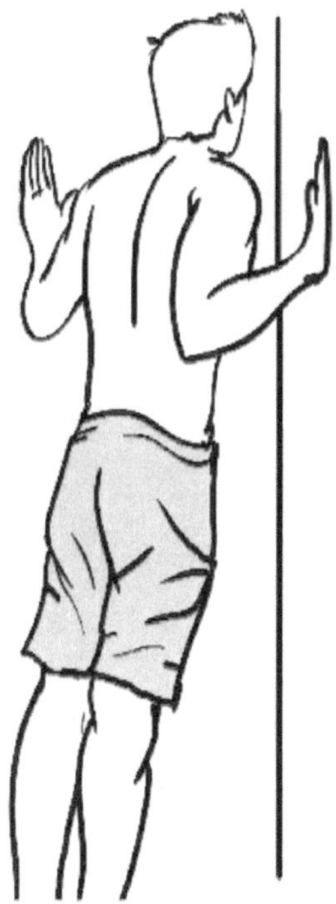

3. Corner Pec Stretch

- Stand a few feet away from the corner of a wall. You will have to adjust how far you stand, depending on your height and the length of your arms.
- Place your palms on either side of the wall at shoulder level.
- Breathe in, and then as you exhale, engage your core and pull them into your back, press your chest into the wall by leaning into it with your whole body.
- Your body should not be bending to accommodate this move. Hold for 30 seconds and repeat three to five times.
- Holding this position results in the chest muscles lengthening.

This stretch targets the pectoralis minor, which is vital in the posture of your upper body. Tight pecs may lead to a hunched back because when they have not been stretched enough, they shrink and pull your shoulders in. It is vital to have good posture when working out and in general. You will not be able to get the best out of your upper body workouts if you do not address posture issues, it is better to prevent this then try and fix it when you already have it.

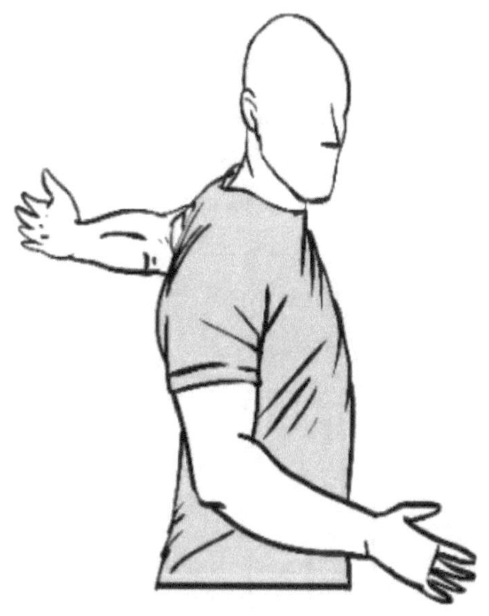

4. Big Turn Back Stretch

- Face a wall and stand as close to it as possible.
- Place your right arm flat against the wall with your palm on the wall. Your arm should be perpendicular to your body and completely straight against the wall.
- Slowly start rotating your torso to the left, leaving your arm stuck against the wall.
- Stop when you feel the stretch in your shoulder and chest. You can continue to deepen the stretch slowly, if you would like more of a stretch, make sure you do not take it too far.
- Hold for about 30 seconds and repeat on the other side.

This stretch helps open up your chest, stretch out your biceps, and loosen up your shoulders. It also has a positive effect on your posture. You will be using all of these muscles for lifting, pressing, and any other upper body workouts.

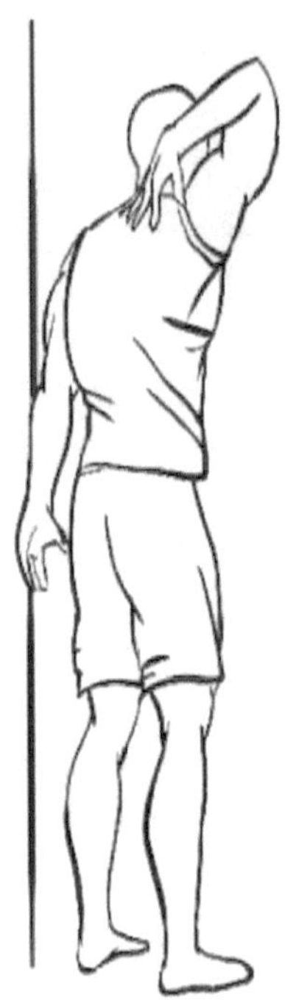

5. Wall Triceps Stretch

- Bend your left arm at the elbow and place the elbow on the wall, slide it up so that it is above your head. Your hand should be behind you, at the center of your back.
- Take your right hand and grab your left wrist.
- Lean into the wall and feel the stretch.
- Hold for 30 seconds and repeat on the other side.

The triceps are used to help move and extend the elbow, and it also plays a role in keeping the shoulder stable. Your whole arm and shoulders will loosen up and be more mobile if you use this stretch.

Most of us have experienced a spine that clicks at some point, the clicking or popping has to do with the general muscle and joint function. There is usually nothing wrong with cracking your back, but it can indicate that you have not been working on or stretching your spine enough. The spine holds up your entire upper body, so we want it to be mobile and functioning correctly. Doing a stretch is a good way of keeping the spine supple, and if done regularly, will hold less tension.

Thoracic Routine

The thoracic region is the region from below your shoulders to above your hips, your abdominal area. This region contains twelve vertebrae and your ribs; all your vital organs are found in this part of the body.

When you work out, your muscles heal and shorten; this happens especially when you sleep. Shortened muscles mean stiff muscles, and this can negatively impact your next workout. To help ease this and help you be in a better position for your next workout, you need to stretch out the thoracic region.

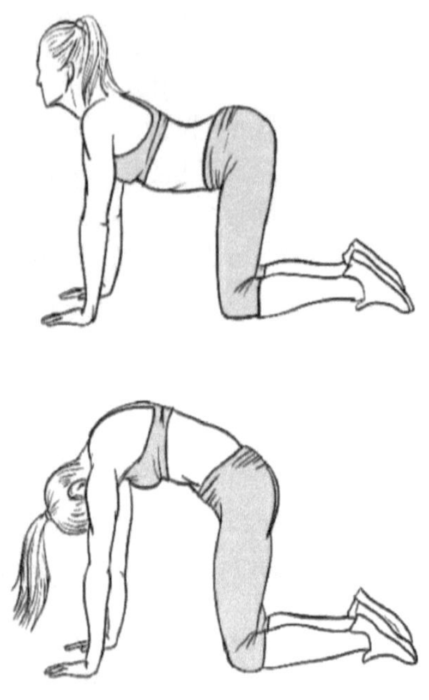

1. Cat-Cow

- Follow the instructions for the Cat-Cow Stretch under the Back and
  Torso routine in chapter 2.

This stretch has been known to improve balance significantly, and it engages
all the vertebrae. It engages the tailbone to activate the root movement of the
spine; this allows the spine to bend more freely. When your spine is more
flexible and has a higher mobility, it will reduce your risk of injuries for
many different workouts.

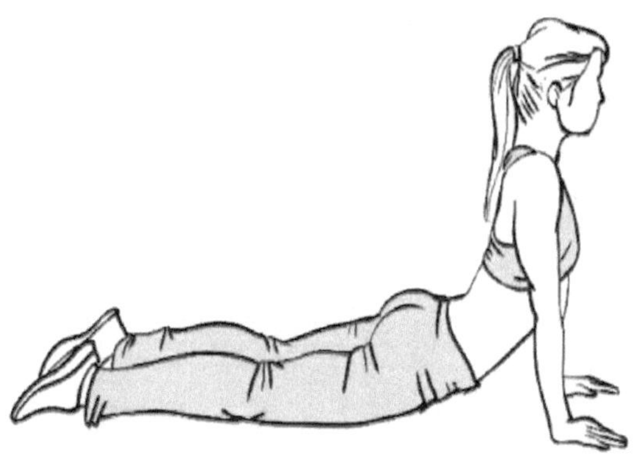

2. The Cobra

- Follow the instructions for the Cobra Stretch under the Back and Torso routine in chapter 2.

The cobra is a spinal stretch that will strengthen your spine. It is also suitable for stretching out the chest, shoulder, and abdomen. Daily activities can impact your spine and spine health, sitting at a desk or even carrying a child causes our spine to bend forward. This can hinder us in many areas, including our fitness, this stretch helps counteract some of the effects of our daily lives.

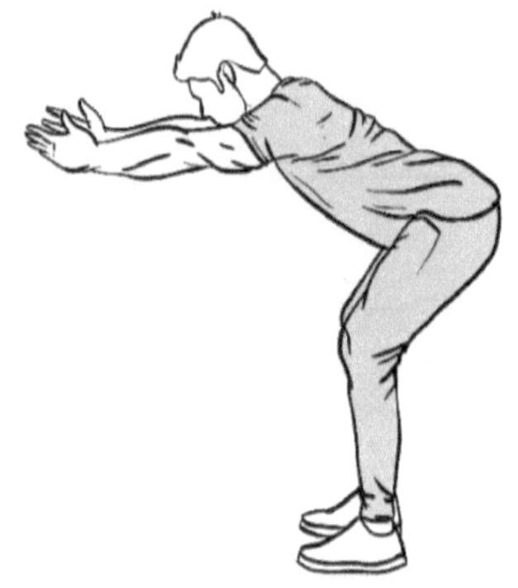

3. The Hip Hinge

- Follow the instructions for the hip hinge under the Back and Torso
  routine in chapter 2.

Bending is part of our general lives, so we need to have a strong core and
lower spinal area. This is also important when it comes to strength training,
deadlifts, kettlebell swings, and many other exercises that require you to have
a strong lower back and core. This stretch strengthens your spine and core so
that you have mobility in these areas.

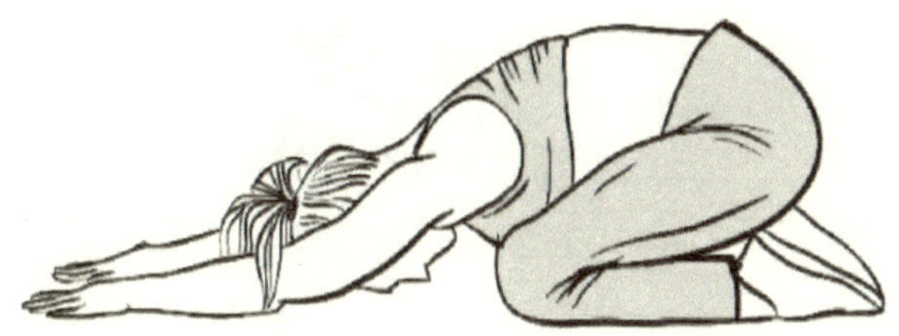

4. Child's Pose

- Follow the instructions for the Child's Pose under the Neck,
  Shoulder, and Chest routine in chapter 2.

Child's pose is incredibly versatile in terms of what body parts it stretches out. It helps with stabilizing the spine and opening up the chest and hips. We tend to have compression in our lower backs because we push our extra weight there instead of engaging our abdominal muscles. This pose helps us release that compression and can make us more conscious of engaging our core.

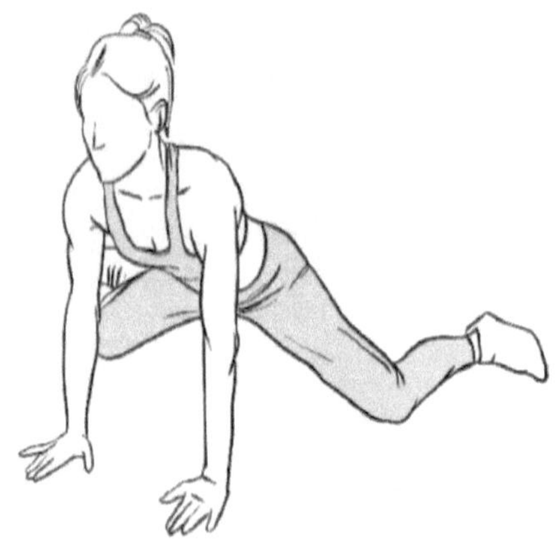

5. The Frog Stretch

- Get down on your hands and knees.
- Turn your feet inwards so that the inner part of the foot is on the floor, and slide your knees apart. They should be wider than your shoulders.
- Drop your hips towards your feet.
- If you can get down onto your forearms instead of on your hands, this will give you a deeper stretch.
- Hold for 30 seconds to 2 minutes.

This stretch works on your groin and adductors, but it also targets your core, which is why it is in this routine. If you have done any kind of exercise or are an athlete of any kind, you will know how important the core is to almost anything you do. Your core muscles are where most of your strength comes from, so having a flexible and robust core will improve your ability in any exercise.

Lower Back and Hips

Building up your flexibility, mobility, and strength in your lower back and hips is the best way to prevent injuries in these areas. A lower back and hip injuries are amongst the most common in the fitness world. Not only is preventing injury important, but strengthening this area helps you get a better lower body workout and upper body workout. This area sits in the middle of your body, and it tends to carry a lot of weight and pressure from exercise and daily activity. Follow this routine to strengthen your lower back and hips.

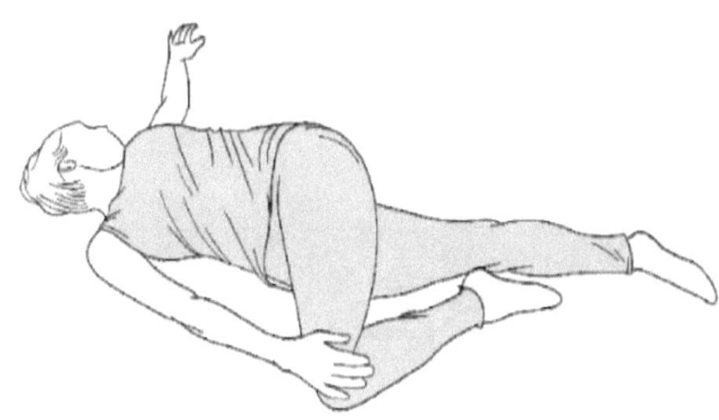

1. Supine Spinal Stretch

- Lay down on your back and bring your right knee up to your chest.
- Take your left arm and bring your right knee down to cross the body
  and land on the left side.
- Stretch out your right arm to the side and turn your head to look at it.
- Hold for 30 seconds and repeat on the other side.

This move helps stretch out your spine, lower back, and it opens up your chest, moving the lower body in a way that it usually doesn't target joints and muscles that are often neglected.

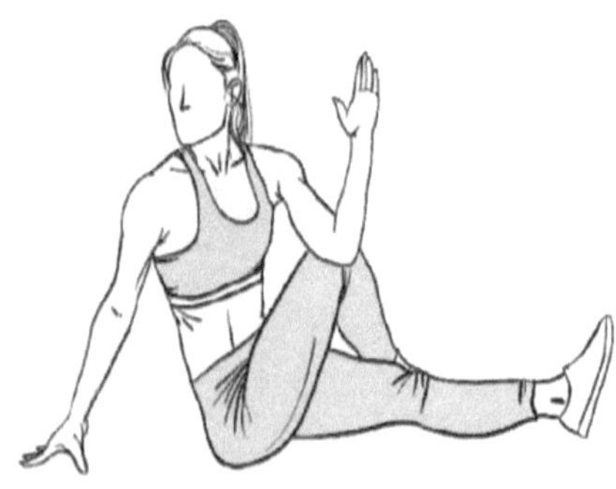

2. Seated Piriformis Stretch

- Sit on the edge of a chair with your back straight.
- Take your left leg and place the ankle on top of your right thigh. Flex

the foot and let it be parallel to the floor.
- Pin down your leg by placing your hand on the ankle and the other hand on the thigh.
- Lean forward and bring your chest into your shin. Go as far as you can to deepen the stretch.
- Keep your back straight at all times.
- Hold for 30 seconds to 2 minutes and repeat on the other side.

This stretch will target the piriformis, glute, and outer hip joints and muscles. These muscles and joints are all important in the movement of the lower body. You will be using them whether you are performing strength training or doing athletic training.

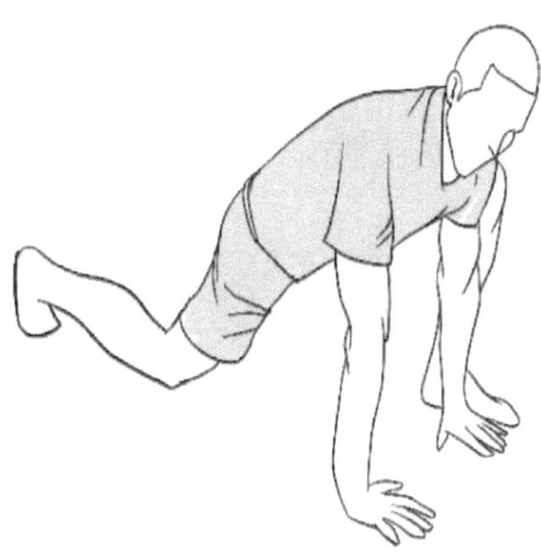

3. The Knight Stretch

- Follow the instructions for the Knight Stretch under the Knees and Thighs routine in chapter 2.

The knight stretch opens up your hips and stretches out your leg muscles; it also stretches your spine and opens up your chest. Stretches like these show you how one move can affect so many different parts of the body. It also shows how connected your body is and why mind-body balance is important.

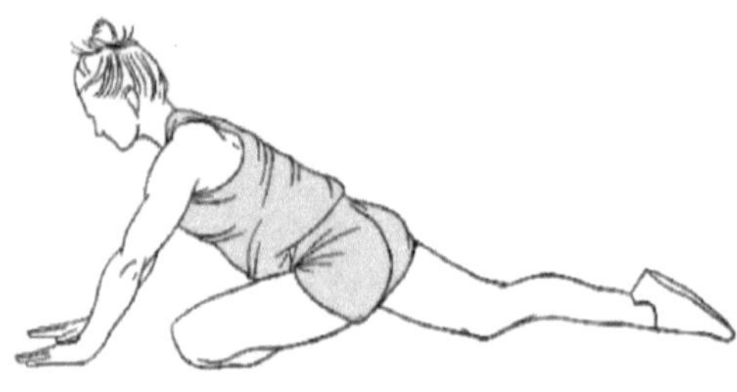

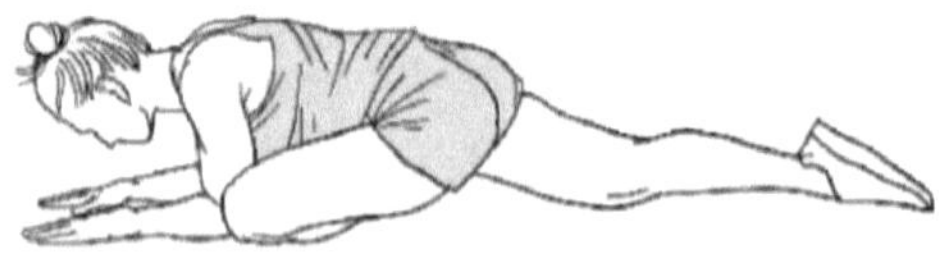

4. Pigeon Pose

- Follow the instructions for the Pigeon Pose under the Hips and Glutes routine in chapter 2.

When you have tight hip flexors, it pulls your pelvis forward, and this has some negative effects on your lower back. Your lower back might have an exaggerated arch, and what this means is that in certain positions or moves, you will feel pain. Loosening up those hip flexors with this stretch will help get a healthier back arch and give you more freedom when you are exercising.

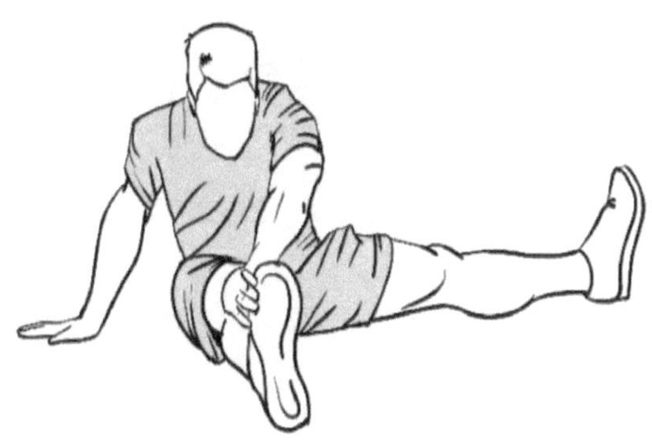

5. The V-Sit

- Sit on the floor with your back straight and your legs open as far apart as you can get them.
- Lean over with your whole body to try and reach your foot. You may not be able to grab your foot; in this case, grab your shin or thigh.
  Push down into your leg until you feel the stretch in your hamstring.
- Hold for 30 seconds and repeat on the other side.

This stretch will help you to measure the flexibility you have in your hamstrings and your lower back. Doing this stretch will allow you to have a wider range of motion in your hips and a stronger lower back.

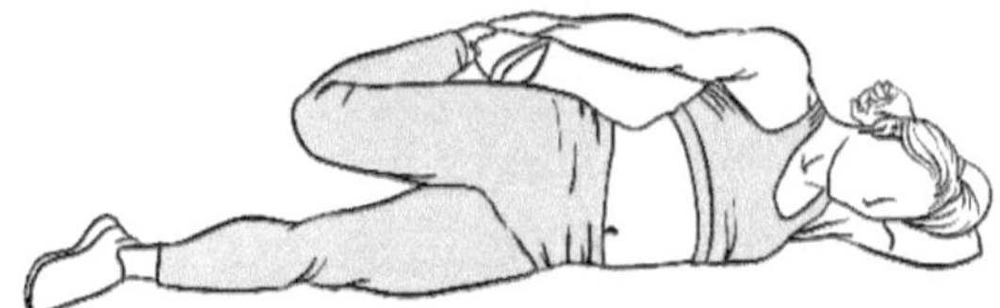

Lower Body

1. Quad Stretch

- Follow the instructions for the Quad Stretch under the Knees and Thighs routine in chapter 2.

This stretch works on not only the quads but also the hips, knee, and other muscles in the leg. This is especially good for strengthening and stretching your legs in preparation for intense lower-body movements. Cyclists,

runners, and people who do yoga all look to this stretch to prepare them for
their exercise and help them cool down afterward.

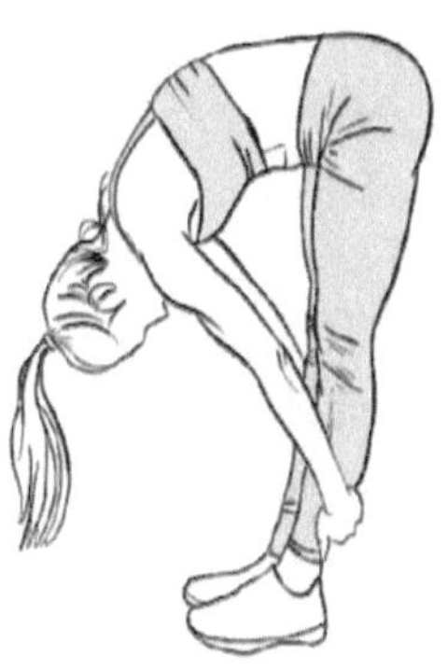

2. Hamstring Stretch

- Sit down on the ground with your legs straight out in front of you and
  your back straight.
- Breathe in and fold your body over your thighs, reach for your feet. If
  you cannot reach your feet, then go as far as you can until you feel the
  stretch in your hamstrings.
- If you want more of a stretch, you can flex your feet.
- Hold for 30 seconds, come back up and shake out your legs. Repeat
  three times.

Hamstring stretches help loosen up the hamstring, and as a result, this gives your body more support. A stringer hamstring will also offer your knees more support when running and performing other exercises.

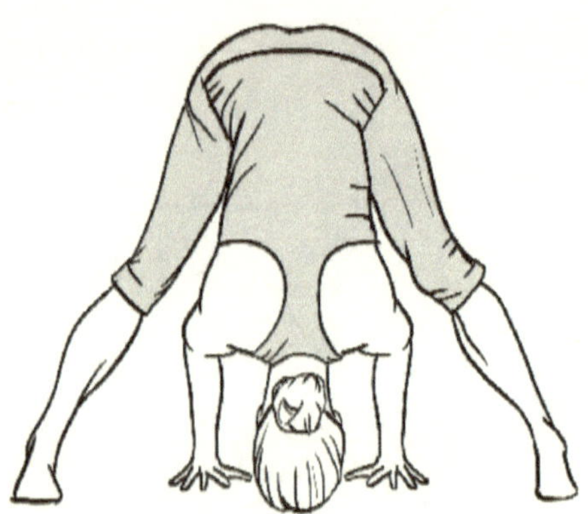

3. Standing Forward Fold

- Stand up with your back straight and feet apart.
- Bend at your hips and bring your body as close to your thighs as you can. Try and keep your knees straight as your reach for the floor with your fingertips. If this is not possible, then reach for your ankles or calves.
- Try and move closer to your thighs with every exhale.
- Hold for 30 seconds to 1 minute.

This stretch will help lengthen the hamstrings and strengthen the knees and thighs. You might also feel something in your calves and hips; this is a stretch that works out most of your lower body.

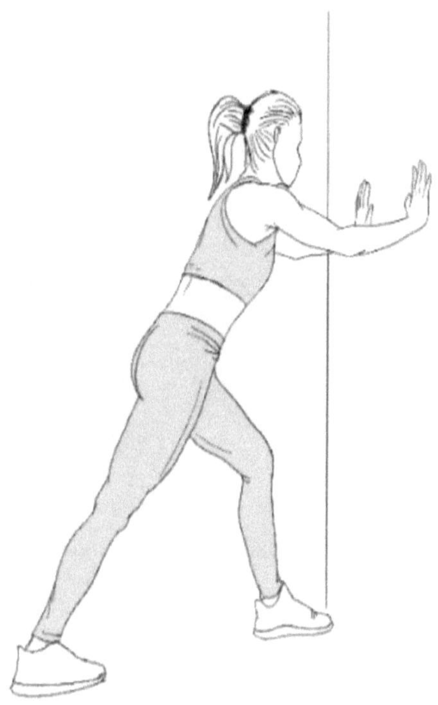

4. Wall Calf Stretch

- Stand a few feet away from a wall.
- Step forward with one leg and leave the other behind. Both feet should be facing forward.
- Hold your hands up against the wall.
- Bend the knee closest to the wall and keep the other leg straight.
- Lean into the wall with your body. Keep both feet planted on the ground. You should feel the stretch in the calf of your back leg.
- Hold for 30 seconds to 1 minute and repeat on the other side.

This stretch will work out your calf but also your Achilles tendon. This means that there will be a wider range of motion, and your lower leg and ankles will be strengthened.

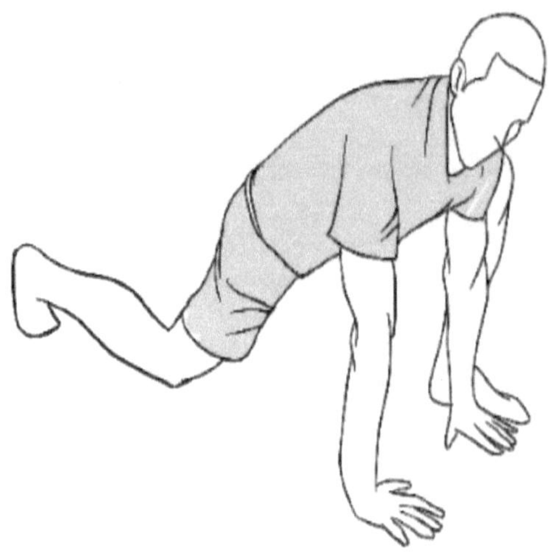

5. The Knight Stretch

- Follow the instructions for the Knight Stretch under the Knees and Thighs routine in chapter 2.

Also, see notes under the lower back and hips routine in this chapter.

THE COOL DOWN: THE ROUTINE TO KEEP YOU, YOUNG

S tretching has so many benefits, not only for your body but also for your mind and your overall well-being. It is a brilliant way to help with injuries and enhance workouts, but we cannot forget the other benefits that come along with it. In general, having excellent flexibility will add to your life, and being more mindful of your stretching can increase your quality of life to a level you would not expect.

THE ROUTINE

Before we jump into the routine, let's focus on meditation and breathing, which are yoga practices, but they extend further than that. These are essential aspects of stretching and improve the way you feel when you are done with the routine and throughout the rest of the day. They help us connect with our bodies and increase how effective our stretches can be.

The importance of yoga is that it does not focus just on the physical body but on the mind as well. What goes on in our mind can affect our bodies, that is why it is so important to be mindful and be able to take control of our thoughts. This is where meditation comes in; meditation helps get the mind-body balance right. It helps us to focus our minds on what is going on in our body, and we can respond to this effectively. Our mind and body are not separate entities, but instead, they work together. This, in turn, will help with everyday movements and control of your emotions, which believe it or not have a huge effect on the pain we feel in our body too. The power to be in control of your mind and your body will lead to a more fulfilling life. This will also be reflected in the response of your body.

Breathing, as we know, is important in general life, but it is essential in stretching. When we focus on breathing, we start focusing on our bodies; this can lead to a lower risk of injury. Breathing will increase our oxygen intake; our muscles need the oxygen to run at their best. Be mindful of when you exhale and inhale, this can also be a tool to help deepen your stretches and reduce the stress that causes knots and tension.

Now let's get into the stretching routine. This routine is excellent for increasing flexibility in your whole body; it was developed by Winderl (2020). Paired with the breathing and meditation techniques we have just spoken about, it is a winning combination for a full mind and body routine.

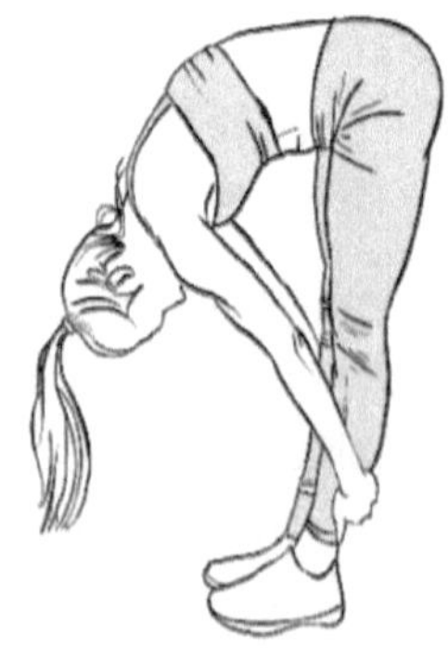

1. Standing Hamstring Stretch

- Start by standing up straight with your feet aligned with your hips.
- Breathe in and fold your body over at the hips, grab the back of your legs at the lowest point you can get it.
- Your upper body should be relaxed.
- Hold for 45 seconds - 2 minutes.

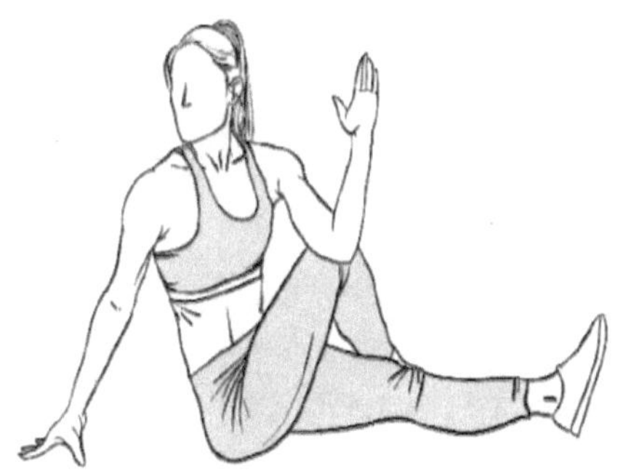

2. Piriformis Stretch

- Follow the instructions for the Piriformis Stretch under the Back and Torso routine in chapter 2.

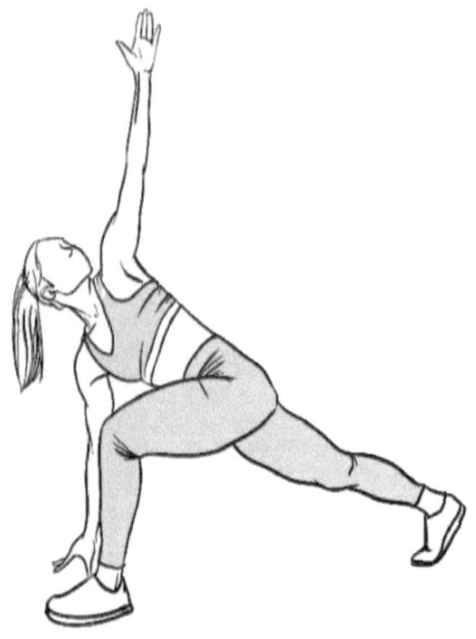

3. Lunge With Spinal Twist

- Follow the instructions for the Lunge With Spinal Twist stretch under the Hips and Glutes routine in chapter 2.

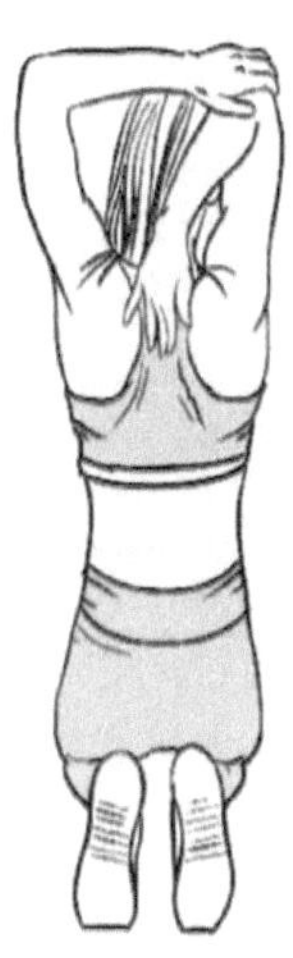

4. Triceps Stretch

- You may stand, kneel, or sit for this stretch.
- Extend your arms above you.
- Bend your arms at the elbow, and touch the center of the top of your back with your hand.
- With your other hand, reach over and grab and pull down gently on the elbow of the bent arm.
- Hold for 30 seconds, repeat on the other side.

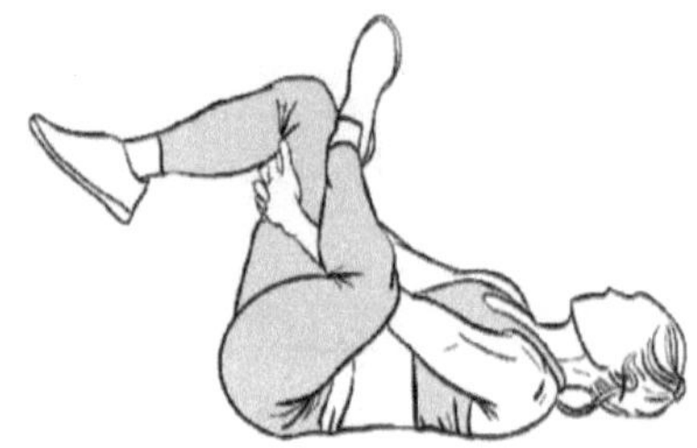

5. Lying Figure 4 Stretch

- Follow the instructions for the Lying Figure 4 Stretch under the Hips and Glutes routine in chapter 2.

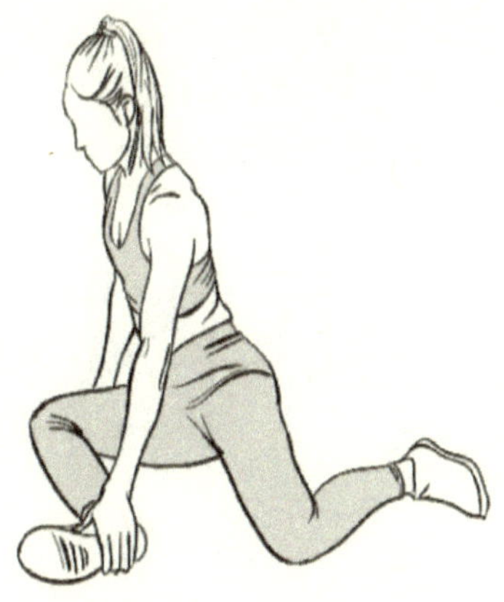

6. 90/90 Stretch

- Follow the instructions for the 90/90 Stretch under the Hips and Glutes routine in chapter 2.

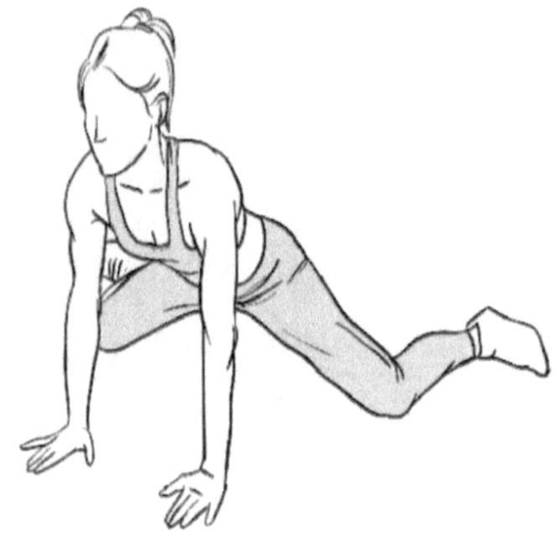

7. The Frog Stretch

- Follow the instructions for the Frog Stretch under the Thoracic
  routine in chapter 4.

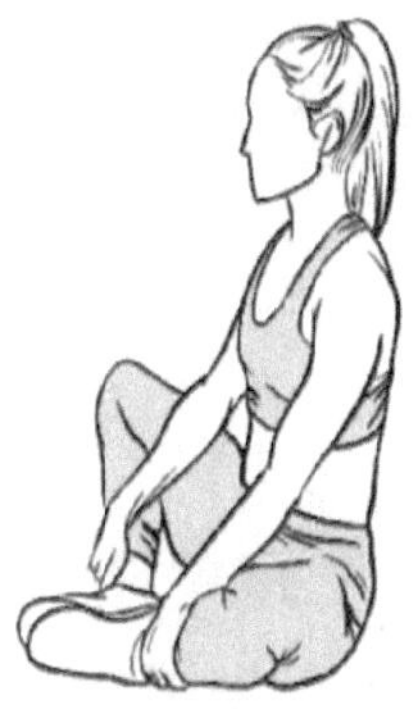

8. Butterfly Stretch

- Sit on the floor with the bottoms of your feet touching.
- Lean over and try to get your head as close to the floor as possible. Push down on your knees with your elbows.
- The closer your feet are to you, the deeper the stretch will be.
- Hold for 30 seconds to 2 minutes.

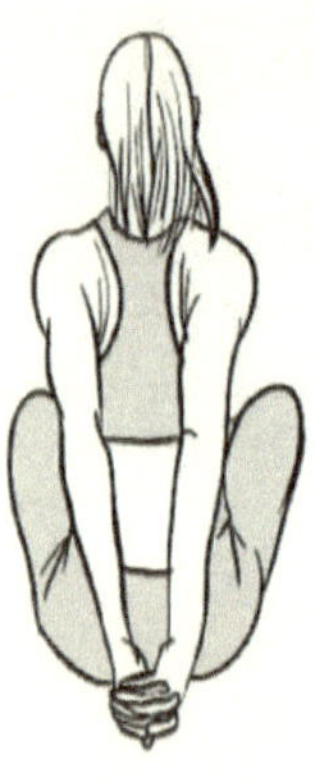

9. Seated Shoulder Squeeze

- Sit down on the ground, bend your knees and have your feet flat on the ground.
- Interlock your fingers behind you.
- Straighten out your arms; you will feel your shoulder blades pulling together.
- Hold for 3 seconds—repeat between five and ten times.

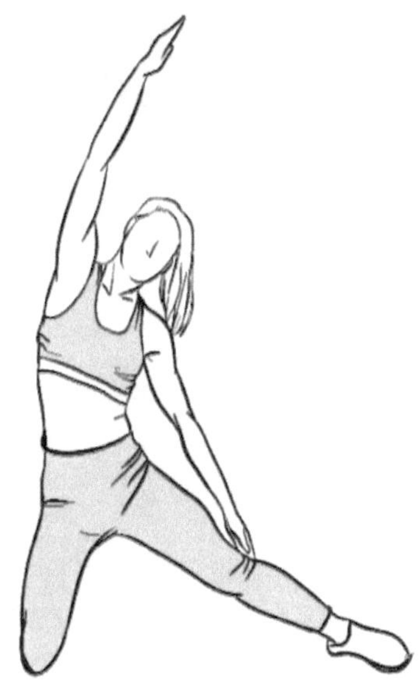

10. Side Bend Stretch

- Kneel on the ground. Keep your back straight.
- Straighten out your right leg to the side.
- Place your right arm on your right leg and lift your left arm in the air.
- Lean your body and arm over to the right.
- Your hips should be facing straight in front of you and your right leg perpendicular to your body.
- Hold between 30 seconds and 2 minutes.

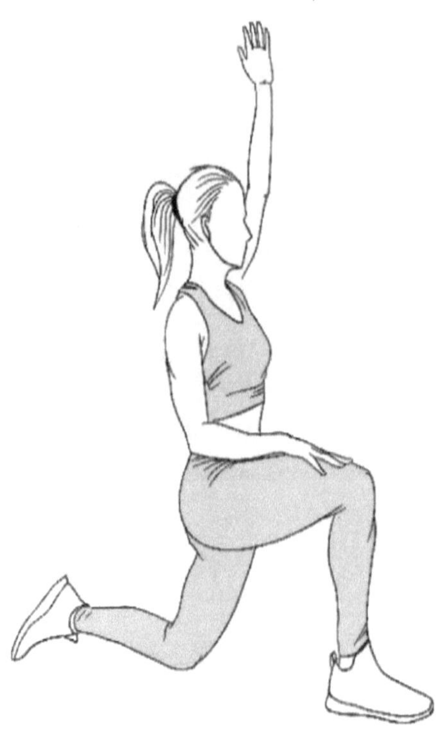

11. Lunging Hip Flexor Stretch

- Kneel on one knee.
- Lean into the leg that is in front of you with your hips.
- If you squeeze your butt, it will give you more of a stretch.
- Hold between 30 seconds and 2 minutes. Repeat on the other side.

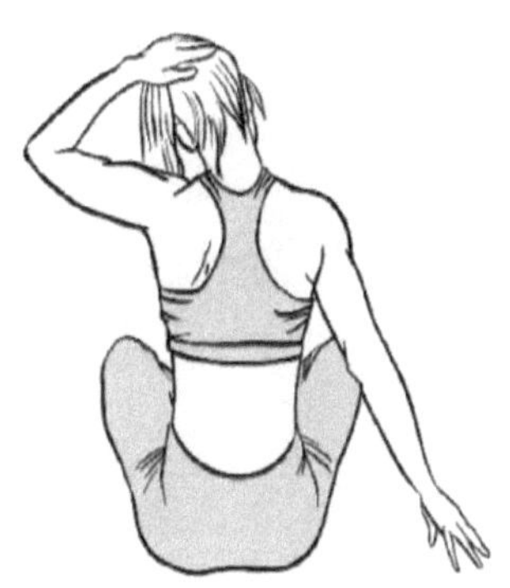

12. Seated Neck Release

- Sit or stand with your back straight.
- Move your right ear towards your right shoulder.
- Take your right hand and slowly pull your head closer to your shoulder.
- Hold between 30 seconds and 2 minutes.

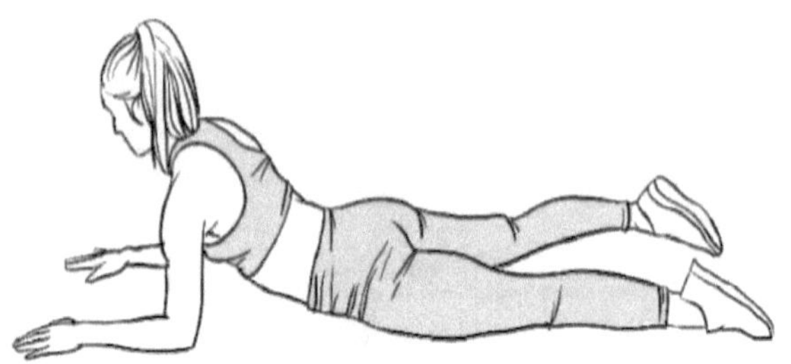

13. Sphinx Pose

- Follow the instructions for the Sphinx Pose under the Back and Torso routine in chapter 2.

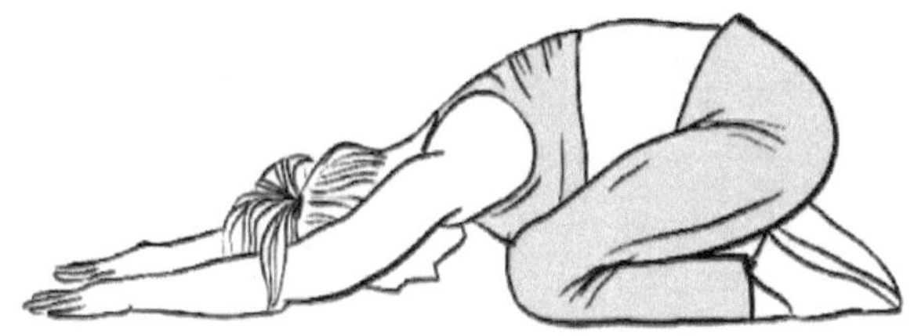

14. Child's Pose

- Follow the instructions for the Child's Pose under the Neck, Shoulder, and Chest routine in chapter 2.

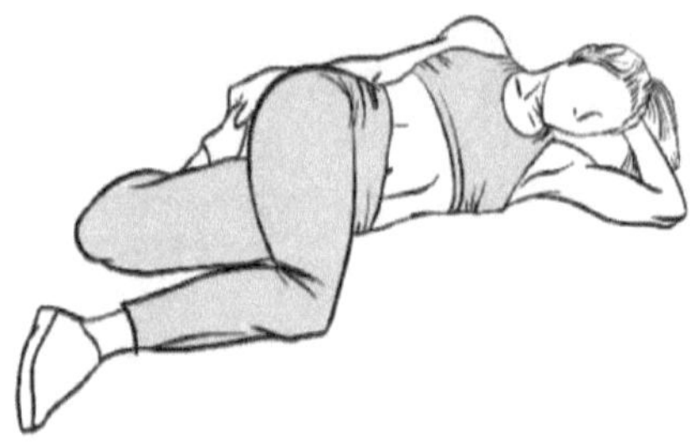

15. Pretzel Stretch

- Lay on the ground flat on your right side. Rest your head on your arm.
- Bend your left leg and bring it up as close to your body as possible.
- Bend your right leg back and grab it with your free arm, pull it up as close to your butt as possible.
- Slowly bring your left shoulder towards the ground, while keeping your torso straight.
- Hold between 30 seconds and 2 minutes. Repeat on the other side.

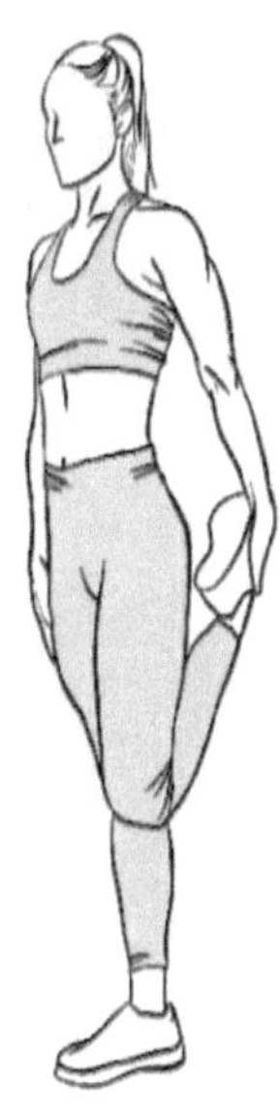

16. Standing Quad Stretch

- Stand up with your back straight and feet together.
- Bend one of your knees back and grab your foot with your hand. Pull the foot towards your butt.
- Do not let your knees separate.
- Squeeze your butt for more of a stretch.
- Hold between 30 seconds and 2 minutes.
- Repeat on the other side.

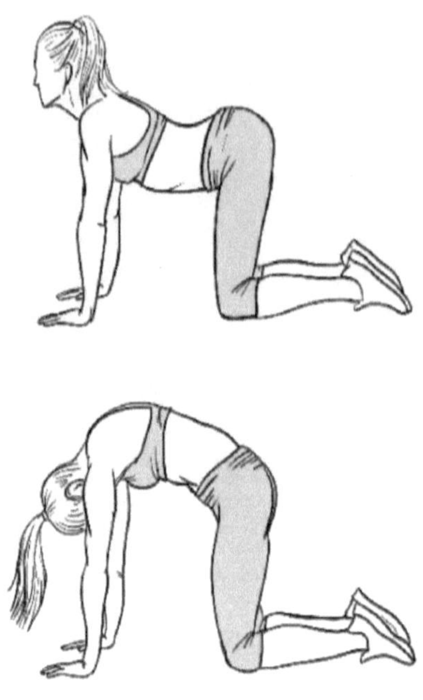

17. Cat-Cow Stretch

- Follow the instructions for the Cat-Cow Stretch under the Back and Torso routine in chapter 2.

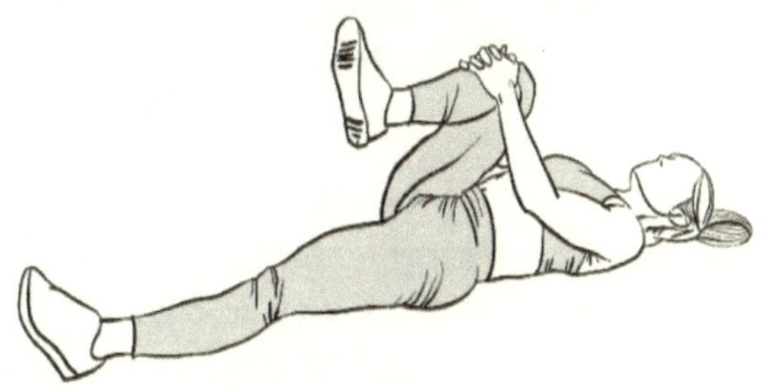

18. Knees to Chest

- Lay down on the ground with your back on the floor.
- Bring your knees up towards your chest.
- Hold onto your shins with your hands and pull them into you.
- Don't allow your lower back to lift off the floor.
- Hold between 30 seconds and 2 minutes.

LIVE A HEALTHY LIFESTYLE

No part of your body runs on its own. Everything is connected and works together for the good or the bad of the entire body and mind. That is why it would not be right to just talk about stretching without mentioning some other aspects that work with stretching to keep you healthy and happy.

We must never forget that no matter how much stretching and exercise we do, if we do not feed ourselves the right nutrition, it might all be in vain. What you eat and how your body performs work side by side. This is why we need to pay attention to what we are putting in our bodies; it can either fuel us or zap our energy. Stick to foods that are high in nutrients, pick whole foods, and always try and incorporate fruits and vegetables into your meals wherever you can. You will feel the difference in your body, in your mind, and your energy levels. Vitamin B is essential within body processes such as energy production.

Sleep is also an important part of a healthy lifestyle. Most people overlook sleep, but it is what will give us energy for the next day. When we sleep, our body repairs itself, and our mind resets itself to prepare for the next day. When we get too little sleep or low quality sleep, we rob our bodies of the opportunity to do this, and before we even get a chance to decide how the day is going to go, we are already on the back foot. If you sleep well, your body will function better; you will be sharper and make better decisions throughout the day. Sleep is one of the main issues I encounter when training clients, and before you work on your fitness and flexibility, getting your sleep right is hugely important.

Give biohacking a try; it can help you discover more about yourself. What your body likes and doesn't like, and how it responds to different patterns and foods. Biohacking is making small changes to your life and lifestyle so that you can see changes in your health and well-being (Jewell, 2019). Much of biohacking is trial and error, or some may describe it as split-testing, but it can help you get a better understanding of your specific body. You could try a diet where you remove one thing and then slowly reintroduce it and see how it makes you feel, or try adding caffeine to your diet as a productivity and energy booster. Try going to bed at different times or having a different bedtime routine and take note of how it affects your sleep. The good thing about biohacking is that you might uncover a secret to a better life that you didn't know before.

When you have a healthy lifestyle, it causes a ripple effect in your life that flows into many areas. Think about it; when you are healthy, you have positive inputs that will respond with positive outputs and responses. You will notice your body thanking you through less pain and your mind thanking you through more emotional control and fewer swings. It affects the way you think because you are more positive and positivity breeds opportunity. You will be more motivated to live better and give more. Other people want to be around happy people. This will vastly improve your relationships and help you to create new ones, stronger ones. Let's not forget how stretching can boost your mood as well; when we stretch, our body releases endorphins, which give us a high and lift our mood. This feeling can last many hours after you have finished stretching and can translate into how you handle situations and people around you.

At the core of this healthy lifestyle is a mind-body balance. We need to have this because it is so important to be healthy all around and not just in one aspect; if we focus too much on one thing, we will not be steady, and it won't be long before we crumble under the pressure of whatever comes our way. Health is made up of pillars of mind and body, and we need to make sure both of them are strong.

It's all well and good to say that you need this balance, but the big question is how to get it. There are actually quite a few things you can do in your life to help you get to a state of overall wellness. Get up and get moving. Sitting down for too long can have negative effects on your body and mind. Aim for 15 minutes of heart elevating activity every day. Do something that feeds your soul, ask yourself where your passion lies, and find a way to integrate that into your life. Treat everyone with kindness, give back, and take the time to slow down and be a part of the world around you and practice gratification. One of the most important ones is to remember to laugh, those same endorphins that are released when you stretch are released when you laugh. These are only a few of the ways you can move towards a mind-body balance, and anything that brings you joy and peace can be added to this list.

There are many facets to health, so remember to explore and pay attention to all of them. Balance is achievable if you take the right steps towards it. It isn't a foreign or make-believe concept but rather something available to all of us. It is your life and your body, and you want to live it the best you can, so whatever that is, make every decision from now in aid of moving in that direction.

YOUR MISSION SHOULD YOU CHOOSE TO ACCEPT IT.......

I need your help; I am new to publishing and working my socks off day and night to try and bring you the best content in my books.

So, your mission from me is that if you enjoyed the book, leave me a quick and honest review. So we can get my books seen by more people and let them know the quality of my books, this is top secret information and we are running out of time.

P.S. if you did not enjoy the book, instead of leaving a negative review, please contact me letting me know why you did not like the content, and I will do my best to address your concerns

Thank you :)

CONCLUSION

Stiffness and lack of mobility is something that many people just silently suffer from purely because they don't know what to do or where to turn to for help. Luckily that does not have to be your story. The stretches and routines in this book have covered every part of the body that no matter where your problem areas are, you are now equipped to handle them head-on.

Taking what you have learned and letting these stretches guide you will be the deciding factor of whether your body and mind reach its full potential. The body is a beautiful thing; it is the case in which our lives are held, so we should want to take care of it. There is no better way to take care of our body than to give it back its flexibility and full range of motion that has been taken away by sedentary lifestyles or unfortunate circumstances.

Whether you want to take the stretches and create your routine or have a specific goal in mind like getting past an injury that is slowing you down, these stretches will help you. As we have discussed, stretching can also help you optimize your workouts, so this is not just for beginners; in fact, you can start at any level and improve wherever you are. Stretching is beneficial to whoever gives it a shot and wants to see what their bodies can do.

Stretching is not only about improving your body and the physical aspects of your life, but it is about adding something to your routine that will help you live a better overall life. The ripple effect of having a good stretching routine implemented in your life is incredible. From having more mobility and freedom to just being in a better mood and having a clearer mind, these are all available to you if you are willing to put in a bit of effort to see your life change for the better.

Give it a shot, and you will not regret it. The fantastic thing is that you do not have to wait months to reap the benefits stretching offers. Your body will start feeling better quicker than you expect, and your emotions and morality will change and become healthier. That is the goal at the end of the day. We all want to be healthier in all aspects of our lives. Stay committed to the process, and your future self will be thanking you.

REFERENCES

AskDoctorJo. (2012, June 22). Shoulder Pain Treatment & Rehab Stretches - Ask Doctor Jo [Video File] Retrieved May 14, 2020, from https://www.youtube.com/watch?v=DJvQ3ZGWUfQ

AskDoctorJo. (2012, June 22). Back Pain Relief with Extension & Rotation Stretches - Ask Doctor Jo. [Video File] Retrieved May 14, 2020, from https://www.youtube.com/watch?v=wgPf9IJiW5s

AskDoctorJo. (2012, October 2012). Pulled Groin Pain Stretches - Ask Doctor Jo. [Video File] Retrieved May 14, 2020, from https://www.youtube.com/watch?v=22tWXwZ2DF8

AskDoctorJo. (2013, March 13). Quadriceps Stretches for Tight or Injured Quads - Ask Doctor Jo. [Video File] Retrieved May 14, 2020, from https://www.youtube.com/watch?v=BhQimqvU1tM

AskDoctorJo. (2013, March 17). Quadriceps Stretches for Tight or Injured Quads - Ask Doctor Jo Retrieved May 16, 2020, from https://www.youtube.com/watch?v=BhQimqvU1tM

AskDoctorJo. (2013, March 18). Achilles Tendon Stretches - Ask Doctor Jo. [Video File] Retrieved May 14, 2020, from https://www.youtube.com/watch?v=vU_FVahd4HI

AskDoctorJo. (2013, March 20). Hip Flexor Stretches & Exercises - Ask Doctor Jo. [Video File] Retrieved May 16, 2020, from https://www.youtube.com/watch?v=7bRaX6M2nr8

AskDoctorJo. (2013, July 4). Hip Pain & Knee Pain Exercises, Seated - Ask Doctor Jo. [Video File] Retrieved May 14, 2020, from https://www.youtube.com/watch?v=4z5W03XutXg

AskDoctorJo. (2016, May 23). Hamstring Strain Stretches & Exercises - Ask Doctor Jo. [Video File] Retrieved May 14, 2020, from https://www.youtube.com/watch?v=x5gunCRsSPU

AskDoctorJo. (2016, July 26). Hand Arthritis Stretches & Exercises - Ask Doctor Jo. [Video File] Retrieved May 16, 2020, from https://www.youtube.com/watch?v=tRnqF-AFFdw

AskDoctorJo. (2017, August 13). Gluteus Maximus (Glute) Strain Stretches & Exercises - Ask Doctor Jo. [Video File] Retrieved May 14, 2020, from https://www.youtube.com/watch?v=Y3T4IedBd4o&t=247s

AskDoctorJo. (2017, August 16). Wrist Tendonitis Treatment for Pain Relief - Ask Doctor Jo [Video File] Retrieved May 14, 2020, from https://www.youtube.com/watch?v=E7vibxI3yZY&t=665s

AskDoctorJo (2017, August 29). Calf Pain or Strain Stretches & Exercises - Ask Doctor Jo. [Video File] Retrieved May 14, 2020, from https://www.youtube.com/watch?v=XibsfBav_04&t=306s

AskDoctorJo (2017, September 13). 10 Best Rotator Cuff Pain Stretches - Ask Doctor Jo. [Video File] Retrieved May 14, 2020, from https://www.youtube.com/watch?v=hd5TY9c1dLE&t=420s

AskDoctorJo (2018, April 2). 5 Best Carpal Tunnel Syndrome Stretches & Exercises - Ask Doctor Jo [Video File] Retrieved May 16, 2020, from https://www.youtube.com/watch?v=Q5G916yCyF0

AskDoctorJo (2019, July 29). 7 Easy Carpal Tunnel Syndrome Treatments - Ask Doctor Jo. [Video File] Retrieved May 16, 2020 https://www.youtube.com/watch?v=FoKUWlKK_Vc

Axtell, B. (2018, February 26). 9 Foot Exercises to Try at Home. Retrieved May 14, 2020, from https://www.healthline.com/health/fitness-exercise/foot-exercises#marble-pickup

Bedosky, L. (2018, October 15). What's the Difference Between Mobility and Flexibility? | Fitness | MyFitnessPal. Retrieved May 11, 2020, from https://blog.myfitnesspal.com/whats-the-difference-between-mobility-and-flexibility/

Bodyfix, M.-. T. O. O. (2020, April 27). How do spiky massage balls work to relieve muscle tension? Retrieved May 13, 2020, from https://www.mybodyfix.co.nz/blog/how-do-spikey-massage-balls-work/

Cavaliere, J. (n.d.). 4 Stretches You Should Be Doing EVERY Morning! Retrieved May 17, 2020, from https://athleanx.com/articles/4-stretches-you-should-be-doing-every-morning

Cronkleton, E. (2020, May 4). 4 Triceps Stretches for Tight Muscles. Retrieved May 17, 2020, from https://www.healthline.com/health/exercise-fitness/tricep-stretches#stretches

Elorreaga, N. (2018, February 4). Give Yourself A Full Body Mobility Assessment! –. Retrieved May 10, 2020, from https://www.nick-e.com/mobility-assessment/

Fischer-Colbrie, M. (2017, July 18). Stretching Improves Athletic Performance and Health. Retrieved May 17, 2020, from https://blog.bridgeathletic.com/stretching-improves-your-health-strength-training

Freutel, N. (2016, December 19). How to Perform a Lacrosse Ball Massage on Sore Muscles. Retrieved May 13, 2020, from https://www.healthline.com/health/fitness-exercise/lacrosse-ball-massage#3

For Care Education and Research (n.d). 15 Best back stretching exercises (with video). Retrieved May 13, 2020, from https://fcer.org/back-stretching-exercises/

Gelles, D. (n.d.). How to Meditate. Retrieved May 16, 2020, from https://www.nytimes.com/guides/well/how-to-meditate

Gupta, A. (2019, November 21). How to perform the Supine Spinal Twist to reduce lower back pain - watch video. Retrieved May 17, 2020, from https://www.timesnownews.com/health/article/how-to-perform-the-supine-spinal-twist-to-reduce-lower-back-pain-watch-video/517968

Hart Osteopathy. (n.d.). Is the Tension Between Your Shoulder Blades Difficult to Reach? This Stretch is for You! Retrieved May 17, 2020, from https://www.hartosteopathy.com/self-hug-stretch.html

Harvard Health Publishing. (2019, September 25). The importance of stretching. Retrieved May 10, 2020, from https://www.health.harvard.edu/staying-healthy/the-importance-of-stretching

Healthwise. (2019, June 26). Wrist: Exercises. Retrieved May 13, 2020, from https://myhealth.alberta.ca/Health/aftercareinformation/pages/conditions.aspx?hwid=ad1518

Jewell, T. (2019, July 5). Guide to Biohacking: Types, Safety, and How To. Retrieved May 17, 2020, from https://www.healthline.com/health/biohacking

Lackowski, R. (2016, June 24). Stretch of the Week: Seated Piriformis Stretch. Retrieved May 17, 2020, from https://www.athletico.com/2016/06/22/stretch-of-the-week-seated-piriformis-stretch/

Lindberg, S. (2020, March 11). Stretching: 9 Benefits, Plus Safety Tips and How to Start. Retrieved May 10, 2020, from https://www.healthline.com/health/benefits-of-stretching

Marin, K. (2015, March 13). The Importance of Breathing in Yoga. Retrieved May 16, 2020, from https://www.yogabhoga.com/blog/importance-breathing-yoga

Mateo, A. (2020, May 11). 4 Glute Stretches You Should Do Every Day to Run Faster and Avoid Injury. Retrieved May 13, 2020, from https://www.runnersworld.com/training/a28708481/glute-stretches/

McGee, K. (2014, May 12). 5 Health Benefits Of Child's Pose. Retrieved May 17, 2020, from https://www.doyou.com/5-health-benefits-of-childs-pose/

McGee, K. (2015, April 10). 25 Simple Ways to Balance Your Mind, Body, and Soul. Retrieved May 16, 2020, from https://www.doyou.com/25-simple-ways-to-balance-your-mind-body-and-soul-17694/

PhysioRoom. (2018, March 15). PhysioRoom's Guide to Foam Rollers. Retrieved May 13, 2020, from https://www.physioroom.com/info/physiorooms-guide-to-foam-rollers/

Physicians Diagnostics and Rehabilitation (n.d.). Cervical Spine Stretches. Retrieved May 13, 2020, from http://www.rosquistchiropractic.net/docs/SpineCarefortheTherapist.pdf

Popsugar Fitness. (2016, September 13). 5 Easy Ways to Stretch Your Calves. Retrieved May 17, 2020, from https://www.self.com/story/best-calf-stretches-running

Reed-Guy, B. L. M. A. L. (2020, February 3). Arthritis. Retrieved May 15, 2020, from https://www.healthline.com/health/arthritis#symptoms

Rizopoulos, N. (2017, April 12). The Benefits of Pigeon Pose. Retrieved May 17, 2020, from https://www.yogajournal.com/lifestyle/hip-connections

Saint Luke's. (n.d.). Supine Hamstring Stretch. Retrieved May 14, 2020, from https://www.saintlukeskc.org/health-library/supine-hamstring-stretch

Seto, W. (2018, November 22). Neck, First Rib Pain & Stiffness: Anterior Scalene Muscle Stretch. Retrieved May 13, 2020, from https://insyncphysio.com/neck-first-rib-pain-stiffness-anterior-scalene-muscle-stretch/

Spotebi. (2017, July 4). Chest Stretch | Illustrated Exercise Guide. Retrieved May 17, 2020, from https://www.spotebi.com/exercise-guide/chest-stretch/

Stelter, G. (2016, December 18). 5 Good Yoga Stretches for Your Arms. Retrieved May 13, 2020, from https://www.healthline.com/health/fitness-exercise/arm-stretches#8

Stretch Relief. (2019, April 9). Is Stretching Good for My Mental Health? Retrieved May 16, 2020, from https://stretchrelief.com/stretching-good-for-mental-health/

Tran, P. (2015a, April 12). How to Do Sphinx Pose in Yoga. Retrieved May 13, 2020, from https://www.yogaoutlet.com/blogs/guides/how-to-do-sphinx-pose-in-yoga

Tran, P. (2015b, April 12). How to Do Wide-Legged Standing Forward Fold in Yoga. Retrieved May 14, 2020, from https://www.yogaoutlet.com/blogs/guides/how-to-do-wide-legged-standing-forward-fold-in-yoga

Thielen, S. (2015, September 17). 5 Chest Stretch Variations. Retrieved May 13, 2020, from https://www.acefitness.org/education-and-resources/lifestyle/blog/5657/5-chest-stretch-variations/

UC Davis. (2014, April 29). Why Stretching is Extremely Important | Student Health and Counseling Services. Retrieved May 10, 2020, from https://shcs.ucdavis.edu/blog/archive/healthy-habits/why-stretching-extremely-important

Ultra Running. (2013, February 8). Benefits of Hamstring Stretches. Retrieved May 17, 2020, from https://www.ultrarunningltd.co.uk/training-schedule/stretching/benefits-of-hamstring-stretches

Winderl, A. C. M. (2018a, January 19). The 7 Best Stretches for Knee Pain. Retrieved May 13, 2020, from https://www.self.com/gallery/best-stretches-for-knee-pain

Winderl, A. C. M. (2018b, December 18). 12 Exercises and Stretches for Shoulder Pain. Retrieved May 13, 2020, from https://www.self.com/gallery/stretches-to-relieve-tight-shoulders

Winderl, A. C. M. (2020, February 3). 12 Hip Stretches Your Body Really Needs. Retrieved May 13, 2020, from https://www.self.com/gallery/hip-stretches-your-body-really-needs-slideshow

Winderl, A. C. M. (2020, May 8). The 21 Best Stretching Exercises for Better Flexibility. Retrieved May 16, 2020, from https://www.self.com/gallery/essential-stretches-slideshow

Yoga Journal. (2017, April 12). Standing Forward Bend. Retrieved May 17,

2020, from https://www.yogajournal.com/poses/standing-forward-bend